22

BITTER MEDICINE

Greed and Chaos in American Health Care

Jeanne Kassler, M.D.

A Birch Lane Press Book
Published by Carol Publishing Group

To Bob

A Birch Lane Press Book
Published by Carol Publishing Group
Birch Lane Press is a registered trademark of Carol Communications, Inc.
Editorial Offices: 600 Madison Avenue, New York, N.Y. 10022
Sales and Distribution Offices: 120 Enterprise Avenue, Secaucus, N.J. 07094
In Canada: Canadian Manda Group, P.O. Box 920, Station U, Toronto, Ontario M8Z 5P9
Queries regarding rights and permissions should be addressed to Carol Publishing Group, 600 Madison Avenue, New York, N.Y. 10022

Carol Publishing Group books are available at special discounts for bulk purchases, for sales promotion, fund-raising, or educational purposes. Special editions can be created to specifications. For details, contact: Special Sales Department, Carol Publishing Group, 120 Enterprise Avenue, Secaucus, N.J. 07094

Manufactured in the United States of America

10 9 8 7 6 5 4 3 2 1

Library of Congress Cataloging-in-Publication Data

Kassler, Jeanne.
    Bitter medicine : greed and chaos in American health care / Jeanne Kassler.
          p.   cm.
    "A Birch Lane Press book."
    ISBN 1-55972-223-1
    1. Medical care—United States.   I. Title.
RA395.A3K365   1994
362.1'0973—dc20   93-43774
                                                       CIP

CONTENTS

PREFACE

ALTHOUGH THE SYNTHESIS of information in this book is mine, I owe a significant debt to the reporters who cover medicine—especially to those who cover the business of medicine. Contained in the details of their reports is the real story of American health care. They have provided many of the critical building blocks for this construct.

I have looked at the business of medicine through the prism of my training as a general internist. To a clinician's eye, it is evident that forces outside the office play an increasingly dominant role in setting medical practice. This book takes a look at the powers that are directing health care from the wings rather than from center stage. Even in the light cast by the nation's debate on health-care reform, many of these players have remained nestled in safe obscurity.

Generations of physicians have been schooled in "Sutton's Law," the heuristic metaphor named for the bank robber Willie Sutton. When asked why he robbed banks, he allegedly said, "Because that's where the money is." The intended lesson was that doctors should think of the obvious diagnoses before they seek the obscure. This book is a variation on that theme. It looks at where the money is—as a way of looking at medicine.

Over the eighteen months that this book was written, both the government and the business of health care changed. Bill Clinton was elected president and Hillary Rodham Clinton headed a task force that pushed reform to the front burner and that delivered the Health Security Act to Congress. On Wall Street, blue-chip pharmaceutical stocks slumped under the pressures of health-care reform while managed-care entities posted impressive gains. Mergers swept health-care businesses, creating behemoths intended to escort us into a healthier future. Insurance companies rushed to recreate themselves as managed-care providers. But while the details change daily, the plot of health care has followed a predictable trajectory—one that began long before the current efforts of reform.

Besides acknowledging my debt to those reporters who cover medicine, especially those at the *Wall Street Journal* and the *New York Times*, I want to thank certain individuals who helped turn this book's concept into reality.

A special thanks to my agents, Deborah Geltman and Gayle Benderoff, and to my editor, Bruce Shostak. They helped nurture the idea into finished manuscript. To the people who trusted a stranger with potentially sensitive information, I extend a thank-you—both to those who wished to remain anonymous and to those who, with their consent, are named in the book.

Like many authors, I owe a large debt to my family. This book could not have been written without their support. But they also served as a constant reminder of life's personal side, where we can let ourselves unwind, where we take our privacy for granted. We have a right to expect that this division between private and public selves will be respected not only by family and friends, but also by everyone involved in our personal medical care.

To my husband, a special thanks for practical as well as emotional support.

INTRODUCTION:
MEDICINE HAS CHANGED

EVEN BEFORE HEALTH-CARE REFORM took center stage during the 1992 presidential campaign, medicine was changing. It had been for decades. But when reformers described what was wrong, they seemed to turn their back on the details of history, on the complicated tale of medicine in the United States since the 1960s. Everyone could agree that the twin issues of rising costs and diminishing access were driving us to change, but fewer people agreed about the root causes.

Reformers spoke with a level of confidence that wasn't shared by many doctors, who were used to dealing with individual patients stranded in the webs of their ailments. Even the hidden voices of Washington analysts, the minds behind the General Accounting Office and the Congressional Budget Office investigations, were more cautious. Things don't always turn out as planned. Small details—like how often a screening test is done—can mean a difference of billions of dollars.

Medicine changed when insurers took over the job of paying medical bills. It wasn't that patients suddenly sought access to free care, it was that massive funding to pay for this care was suddenly available. The age of third-party payers unleashed the health industry's entrepreneurial zeal. Hospital chains sprouted, medical device companies grew, physicians switched from talking to patients to doing procedures on them. Altruism was no longer the driving force. High technology, with its advances and costs, replaced the more modest achievements of earlier decades.

We got a lot in return, but at a very high price. After 1965, when Congress passed Medicare and Medicaid, health-care costs started to increase at double-digit rates. Health insurers—businesses, government, and insurance companies—eventually balked at the unforeseen and uncontrolled tab. Each had its own strategy of cost containment, whether that was by shifting costs, cutting fees, or scrutinizing medical decisions. There were end-less maneuvers, none of which were aimed at controlling system-wide costs.

By 1993, when President Clinton's task force made health reform prime-time news, industry trends had already started to reshape the practice of medicine. Consolidation was everywhere. The "Wal-Martization" of America had spread to medicine. Even solo practitioners, the equivalent of mom-and-pop stores, were not what they seemed. Many were linked to managed-care networks controlled by industry giants like Prudential or Aetna. And corporations like PhyCor and Pacific Physician Services were buying doctors' practices. Neither patients nor doctors had pivotal roles in setting the health-care agenda.

Although selling health reform to the American public was pegged to selling health security, reformers were still unwilling to admit that unless we realistically controlled costs for the long haul, any security would be transient. The cost debate focused on politically prudent issues like doctors' incomes and pharmaceutical profits. Politicians held fast to the idea that we would need to sacrifice nothing, we would merely eliminate inefficiency. They sidestepped the fact that almost half the increase in health-care costs over the past decade was traceable to two factors having nothing to do with health care—general inflation and demographic changes. The politicians focused on administrative waste and industry fraud which, although consuming billions, were in fact not enough to allow for painless savings.

Reformers avoided the nettlesome question of limiting access to high-cost, high-tech medicine because it raised the specter of deliberate rationing—as opposed to the haphazard rationing we have now. But the volume and intensity of medical services accounted for nearly one third of the rise in health-care costs and, at least in the medical press, were targeted as the most obvious places to look for cost savings.

Some of the revenue that reformers talked about had the aura of funny money. Politicians talked about lowering costs by increasing access to preventive care. But studies don't back their claims that prevention necessarily saves money. Yes, it is cheaper (and certainly more humane) to treat someone's hypertension in the office than to wait for them to wind up in the emergency room with a stroke. But universal screening for hypertension, treating all patients who need drug therapy, monitoring them for a lifetime, and coping with drug side effects is costly.

Reformers counted on increased tax revenues from businesses that would be more profitable once their health costs went down. But what about taxes lost when former health-care workers hit the unemployment lines? The health-care industry had been a source of jobs in an era of shrinking employment, gaining nearly 800,000 jobs in 1991, a time in which 663,000 jobs were lost in the United States. By 1992, health-care employment topped 10 million, an increase of 43 percent in four years—and that 10 million didn't include those who worked in the insurance, pharmaceutical, or medical equipment and supplies industries. Of the ten occupations expected to grow the fastest in the next decade, six were health-related, according to the Bureau of Labor Statistics. One seventh of the nation's economy was tied up in health care. Surely, the price of real health-care reform would mean job losses.

This wasn't a reason not to cut health employment, only a note of caution when doing the calculations of cost savings. Health-care employment had reached absurd dimensions. A catalog of adult education courses advertised "Careers in the Medical Industry," including such courses as "Start a Home-Based Medical Billing Business" from which you can "earn $75,000 to $150,000," "Basic Medical Billing," and "Basic CPT/ICD Coding"—"an area that is growing by leaps and bounds." The complexity of health care made billing for medical services more profitable than providing them.

Another hidden cost of reform was the effect on our trade balance. The output of U.S. pharmaceutical, medical equipment, and medical supply firms makes up nearly half of their industries' production worldwide. These businesses spawned a $3.7 billion trade surplus in 1991, a time in which the country was running a $66.7 billion trade deficit. And the Congressional Budget Office didn't support the view that health-care costs hidden in sticker prices were making other U.S. products—like cars—less competitive.

Although doctors' earnings and pharmaceutical profits got repeated press, reformers were slow to look at the inherent conflict of a system in which businessmen got extremely rich while the rest of us tightened our belts. The chairman of Hospital Corporation of America received $127 million in 1992. *Business Week*'s list of the twenty top-paid CEOs in 1991 listed five executives in the health-care business. A snapshot view of only five companies over six months, gleaned from the *Wall Street Journal*'s tracking of insider trading, showed more than $1 billion in stock transactions by company insiders. In April 1992, Leonard Abramson, the president of U.S. Healthcare, the nation's largest investor-owned HMO, sold stock worth $9,421,000—estimated to be only 10 percent of his holdings. In May, Jeremy Welsh, an officer of Pharmaceutical Markets Service, sold more than $15 million worth of stock, said to be only 13 percent of his holdings. Martin Gerstel, an officer of the biotechnology firm Alza, sold shares worth $6,304,000, which represented 40 percent of his holdings. The same month, Leon Hirsch, chairman of the medical supply firm U.S. Surgical, sold $12,785,000 worth of stock, or 5 percent of his holdings. Two officers of the company also sold nearly $8 million worth of stock in May. In July, Hirsch sold additional shares worth more than $15 million, and an officer sold shares worth more than $13 million. In September a director of the health maintenance organization United Healthcare sold nearly $21 million worth of stock. Stratospheric profits were okay in health care—as long as you worked on the business side.

As the crises in health care push us to reform, we have lost sight of the records of the three main players that have seized the mantle of health-care reform. We should look at the insurance industry, big business, and government and at the compassion and fiscal responsibility that they have shown over the years.

The insurance industry has reinvented itself. Hard-nosed businessmen once sought to exclude sick patients, claiming that was the best practice to ensure affordable insurance for the majority of policyholders. Now, recast as guarantors of managed care, they promise to deliver comprehensive care to all. Comforting television and print commercials assure us that the new insurance industry will have a warm embrace.

Big businesses broke their promises to provide health insurance for retirees and grossly underfinanced their pension plans. Today, more than $45 billion in private retirement funds are underfunded, dominated by the auto, airline, and steel industries. General Motors, a corporation that has been in the vanguard of those seeking to control health-care spending, accounts for more than $17 billion of these underfunded benefits. If these retirement plans went bust, taxpayers would pick up the tab—either directly for those plans that are guaranteed by the Pension Benefit Guaranty Corporation or indirectly because retirees would be forced to rely on publicly funded entitlement programs. Taxpayer liability could grow to rival that of the savings and loan crisis and require billions of dollars. Yet we assume that these same businesses will propose financially sound plans for health-care reform.

The federal government has also had a questionable financial legacy, although, unless it goes broke, it has a better record of keeping promises. Its financial projections routinely miss the mark by huge sums, and it has underfunded its own pension plans even more than big business has—by more than $1 trillion. Within the next fifty years the pension liability of the military alone is expected to grow from over $11 billion to nearly $300 billion.

Also lost in the debate on reform are subtle questions that are not about cost or access. They concern society's values. What we do outside the health-care system may affect our health more than what we do inside. Some studies suggest that those industrialized countries like Japan and Sweden with the smallest income differentials have the best health outcomes. But in the United States, the difference between low and high earners has grown steadily wider. Whereas top CEOs earned 35 times the wage of the average worker in the 1970s, they earned 120 times the average worker's salary in 1990. The CEOs who cry loudly for lowering health-care costs would be unlikely to do so at the expense of those pay differentials.

We cite our infant mortality statistics as a failure of health care. Worldwide, we rank in twenty-second place. But more than one fifth of our children are growing up in poverty. The number of single working mothers reached nearly 6 million in 1991, almost triple the number of twenty years before. Since single mothers often lack good housing, health insurance, adequate day care, and child support from absent fathers, their children are at risk. And it's not just children who are falling from economic grace. Ten percent of Americans were on food stamps in early 1992, a record high. A study by social scientists at Fordham University found that our country's overall sense of well-being in 1990 hit the lowest point since the annual study was begun in 1970.

When we eye reform, we should also look at some of the hidden consequences of proposals. Computerizing medical records has been hailed as a major way to cut administrative costs. But it paves the way for a massive breach of privacy. The Hippocratic oath states that "whatsoever I shall see or hear in the course of my profession, as well as outside my profession in my intercourse with men, if it be what should not be published abroad, I will never divulge, holding such things to be holy secret." But managed health care and electronic highways make the issue moot. One managed pharmacy plan sent a doctor a questionnaire about a patient's pharmaceutical use over the past year. When the physician called the plan administrators to inquire whether they had a signed release, they said that the patient's union—the basis of his insurance—had a general release. They said they would forward a copy of the release, but never did. When the doctor asked the patient whether he had signed a release, the patient angrily denied that he had ever done so.

Although managed care has been purported to deliver cost-efficient care, policy experts are not so sure. Not only are the financial benefits questionable, but managed care's effect on doctor-patient relationships has yet to emerge. Too few people wonder how doctors will be able to behave in a system in which their income depends directly on profit-driven companies that have the power to put them out of business. When PruCare, Prudential's managed-care plan, sent its participating New York physicians a contract in the summer of 1993, it stipulated that primary-care doctors could not stop taking new PruCare subscribers until they had 500 PruCare patients. For a doctor with an average panel of 1,500 patients, that meant PruCare could control one third of his income. Although the company later told recalcitrant doctors that they could close their panels with fewer PruCare patients, such hardball tactics were the wave of the future. If doctors object to clinical policy, how far will they go under these circumstances?

As we move toward reform, we should remember the quip: "There are three kinds of lies: lies, damned lies, and statistics." Analysts can choose the numbers that support their views. We have to be wary of opting for the solution that is politically expedient but doesn't grapple with the real issues.

What follows is a portrait of U.S. health care, in all its unsettling complexity. It is a look at the trade-offs that we have made. It examines the gap between our perceptions of health care and the reality. By looking at how health-care players have acted over the past decades, it offers a glimpse of what we can expect from them under reform.

PART ONE

CHIEF COMPLAINT AND HISTORY

ONE OF THE FIRST LESSONS a student is taught in medical school is to take a good, detailed history from a patient. A correct diagnosis can be made 75 to 90 percent of the time simply by listening to the patient and asking key questions. No fancy lab work, not even the physical exam. Just eliciting the portrait of an illness.

The first goal is to have the patient narrate his "chief complaint," the symptom that made him seek medical care. This chief complaint may be the real problem—or a red herring. But the physician's first task is to bring the chief complaint into focus, to extract those details that turn an amorphous story into the description of an illness. If the doctor cannot immediately define the illness, at least he should be able to gauge its severity.

For example, someone comes into the office because of abdominal pain. The doctor's questions aim to lead to a specific diagnosis, like appendicitis, pancreatitis, or an ulcer. By asking specific questions, he analyzes the situation. When did the pain start? (Pain that started recently is more likely to progress rapidly than pain that's been plaguing someone for many years.) Does the pain wake the patient up at night? (If it does, it's more likely to be serious than pain that subsides during sleep.) Has the patient lost weight unintentionally? (If he has, the illness is probably ruining his appetite or impeding the absorption of food—both are serious problems.) Is there a family history of abdominal problems, like cancer or colitis? (Some diseases tend to run in families, and although the illness may be relatively rare—or rare in a young person—it should be considered in a family member.) Is the pain worse after eating? (Specific diseases, such as gallstones or pancreatitis, have characteristic features such as the timing of the

1

pain or positions that alleviate the pain.)

As the doctor follows the story, his mind's eye traces the diagnostic possibilities. He is developing the "differential diagnosis"—a list of possibilities triaged by probability.

Just how quickly a doctor moves on a situation depends on how serious he thinks it is and also on his reading of what the patient wants. Some patients want a definitive diagnosis immediately, others prefer to tolerate uncertainty in the hope that the malady will pass with a minimum of tests and medications. Some patients send out signals that they're worried about a serious illness but that the physician should lead the way gingerly. Some doctors feel that their job is to hunt down the disease and that others can do the hand-holding. There are different ways of working through a diagnostic tree, tailored to both the patient and the physician.

But this fundamental way of looking at illness, of viewing it through the prism of a differential diagnosis, seems lost when it comes to understanding what's ailing medicine today. The thought process that lies at the heart of medicine has been discarded when it comes to understanding health care.

Many analysts of our medical system have vested interests and political agendas that make them unable to ask the fundamental questions: what went wrong and when did it go wrong? They have vested interests in the answers.

The problems of our health-care system are multiple and interrelated. Most are serious enough that each could be seen as a "chief complaint."

Perhaps the only point of agreement among critics and enthusiasts is that the United States is medicine's technological mecca. Someone may not have access to the latest procedure or he may be the beneficiary of a high-tech procedure that has no proven track record, but—as they say in the commercials for the yellow pages of the regional phone company NYNEX—if it's out there it's in here.

While the rapid diffusion of high-tech medicine has prompted enthusiasts to tout our system as the best in the world, more and more Americans complain that it is the system that ails them—even when they are physically well. Health-care angst is spreading.

What is wrong?

CHAPTER 1

Costs—Headed Higher

THE "CHIEF COMPLAINT" of our system is its cost and its staggering rate of growth. Patients used to go to the doctor, wait for the
bill, and then send a check. Payment was a leisurely affair. Now
everyone is on edge. When patients call to make their first
appointment, receptionists quote fees on the phone. When they
arrive at the front desk, signs warn that payment is expected at the
time of the visit. And if they need to be admitted to the hospital
(on a nonurgent basis), the first stop is the billing department,
which demands proof of insurance and, sometimes, a deposit.

Although the following case is unusual, it illustrates a peculiarly American feature of the high cost of health care, of our
technologically intensive, no-holds-barred system. An eighty-
seven-year-old woman with heart disease and diabetes was hospitalized because she had become increasingly short of breath over
the previous day. Several days later, after her condition deteriorated, she was transferred to the hospital's intensive care unit,
where both her private physician and the director of the intensive
care unit supervised her care.

For nearly six months, she remained hospitalized, most of the
time in the intensive care unit. When her private physician
explained to the family that her chances of survival were slim,
they fired him. When the ICU director did the same, they
threatened to kill him if—not when—the patient died.

The daily cost of the woman's ICU bed was more than $2,000.
But this cost did not include private physicians, specialist consultations, medications, laboratory tests, X-rays, cardiograms,
blood transfusions. And no patient in an ICU merely gets a bed.
For months, the patient used a Clinitron bed, a mechanical bed
that rocks back and forth, specially designed to prevent pressure
sores. The bed, rented from an out-of-state company, added $45

3

per day. Each day that she was on a respirator, her care cost an additional $350. Every time she had a cardiac arrest, it cost $1,600 to restock the code cart, the cart that is wheeled to the bedside loaded with medications used for cardio-pulmonary resuscitation. Each of the more than 40 units of blood she received cost $90. Every chest X-ray cost $125, every cardiogram cost $60—like most ICU patients, she had almost daily chest X-rays and ECGs. She had frequent blood and urine tests, often several times a day. She required oral nutritional supplements, regulated by nutritionists. When these failed to sustain her, surgeons inserted special catheters to feed her intravenously.

Given the quantity of medications, including antibiotics, cardiac drugs, and antiulcer drugs, even the inexpensive ones added up. But many of her drugs were expensive. The antibiotics amikacin and imipenem cost $140 and $65 a day. Some days, she had both. Every day, she was given insulin and heart medications.

Medicaid, her hospital insurer, paid the hospital tab. But it paid only a fraction of the cost. By the time she died, 168 days after admission, her hospital costs totaled $387,887.04. Medicare, her insurer for physician costs, picked up an unknown tab for the multiple specialists who saw her and for her primary doctor, who had advised against the aggressive care.

The hospital, already hundreds of millions of dollars in debt, absorbed almost $250,000 in unreimbursed expenses. In 1991, this hospital spent $50.5 million, or nearly 10 percent of its costs, on the 732 patients who were admitted to its intensive care units. The following year, costs jumped to nearly $56 million for 710 patients.

The prolonged hospital stay and the death threats were unusual, but the intensity of service and its futility were not. Lying in the beds next to the woman were others who also suffered irreversible diseases: a ninety-two-year-old woman with a chest tumor, an eighty-three-year-old man with cardiovascular collapse, and a sixty-three-year-old man with end-stage Parkinson's disease who could not move or speak. Of eighteen patients in the ICU that day, the ICU director estimated that only six were appropriate admissions. Only one out of three patients had a potentially reversible disease. That didn't mean that one out of three would survive or emerge in good health, only that one out of three stood to benefit from treatment that cost roughly $3,000 a day.

Daily, year in and year out, similar scenarios are repeated all across the nation in our country's roughly 100,000 intensive-care-unit beds at an annual cost of nearly $50 billion. One survey found that half of all ICUs had at least one "chronic" patient. If we eliminate those intensive care units devoted to caring for children, we find that nearly 60 percent of the beds are occupied by patients over sixty-five years of age.

Although health-care costs have increased at double-digit rates since the mid-1960s, it is their share of the gross domestic product that has skyrocketed in recent years. We spent only 5.3 percent of our GDP on health care in 1960. But health-care costs as a percentage of our total economic output hit double digits by the mid 1980s, and they are expected to reach 19 percent of GDP by the year 2000 if we let our current system continue. In thirty years, we went from spending $27 billion a year on health care to spending more than $750 billion. By 1993, we spent more than $942 billion on health care, or more than 14 percent of our total economic output, according to the Commerce Department. The sum is projected to top $1 trillion in 1994.

The absolute numbers are staggering, but they don't really register with those more accustomed to their own budgets than national budgets. The leap from thinking in thousands of dollars to thinking in billions requires a stretch of the imagination like fathoming the sun's temperature. It hardly seems real.

But some facts put the abstract into perspective. At the current rate of growth, a family of four could be spending $30,000 a year on medical care by the late 1990s—more than they would be paying for food, clothing, transportation, and housing combined. States have begun to spend more on Medicaid than on colleges and universities. Medicine is becoming a sinkhole that threatens to overshadow all other demands and pleasures of life. And the more we spend, the less secure we feel. Roughly 39 million Americans don't have health insurance. If we provided insurance for them, some experts project that health care would cost an additional $12 billion to $27 billion each year. Those of us who are insured see cautionary tales everywhere. We understand that losing our job or getting sick is all that it might take to enter the ranks of the uninsured.

When a patient describes his chief complaint, one of the doctor's first questions is "When did it start?" He's fishing for a cause, since timing is often a clue to cause. If a patient says that his stomach feels bloated whenever he eats cheese or drinks a lot of milk, it doesn't take a diagnostic genius to think of lactose intolerance. If the patient adds that he first noted the discomfort five years ago but that nothing much has changed, he's told him that his current digestive problem isn't due to a rapidly progressive cancer.

What's noteworthy about health-care costs is that they started to accelerate in the mid-1960s, when the federal government did two things. It created Medicare and Medicaid, the federal insurance plans for the elderly and the poor. A look at health expenditures between 1960 and 1991 shows that double-digit growth started in 1965, the year that Medicare and Medicaid became law.

The other move was a congressional mandate in the early 1960s to increase the number of physicians significantly. Instead of 140 doctors for every 100,000 Americans, there were eventually 250 doctors for every 100,000 Americans. Since physicians generate 75 percent of health-care costs—not because of their incomes, but because they order further care—a 70 percent gain in the number of doctors was certain to fuel medical costs.

Understanding the timing is critical, not just to making us wary of the unforeseen consequences of government acts, but also to letting us see that some factors blamed for our high costs existed long before the current fiscal crisis developed. The incentives of fee-for-service medicine, in which doctors are paid for each activity, are often cited. But physicians always practiced fee-for-service medicine in the United States, and they continue to do so in many countries, such as Canada, Japan, and Germany, that have done a much better job controlling costs. Solo practice, which lacks economies of scale, is also blamed, but it, too, existed before costs skyrocketed and coexists with price moderation in other countries.

Medicare and Medicaid (along with private insurance) provided an unrestricted source of funds from an anonymous third-party payer: the federal government. They severed the connection between paying for and receiving care and let loose a frenzied rate of growth. Doctors were described as pigs at the trough by a former head of the Institute of Medicine. But the opportunity was too good to be left only to physicians—there were others waiting to feed.

The commercial potential of the medical market, fueled by private as well as public insurance, was an incentive for the growth of high-technology medicine, for an aggressive medical arms race. And the costs of technology could rise at extraordinary speed. In 1985, when Medicare first approved payments for magnetic resonance imagers—a very expensive and sophisticated alternative to X-rays—there were only 200 machines. By 1986, there were 2,000 MRIs. In 1990, Medicare paid $237 million for outpatient MRI scans—that was $200 million more than it had paid four years earlier. It was a boon for radiologists and MRI manufacturers.

Technology was the engine of medical cost inflation, running on third-party fuel. A study of Medicare expenses from 1985 through 1988 found that procedures—doing something to patients rather than just talking to them—accounted for 37 percent of all expenditures. During the same four-year period, the costs of advanced imaging, such as CAT scans and MRIs, increased nearly three times faster than the overall 12.3 percent growth rate. The study found that "evaluation and management services [e.g., office visits] were not major contributors to the growth in Medicare expenditures." The miracles of technology had a dark side— you had to pay a lot for them. We had created the core of the U.S. system—a financially incendiary mix of anonymous funding, high technology, and corporate opportunity. Unlike other industries, the modern health-care industry was never constrained by the reality of market forces in the United States.

Amid the criticism of costs, we sometimes lose sight of the fact that many of today's services are a vast improvement over what came before. Diagnostic tools are quicker and safer. CAT scanners replaced pneumoencephalography for diagnosing brain tumors. The old procedure, in which air was injected to outline brain structures, was painful and caused severe headaches. Screening tools are more widespread and accurate. A study by the Centers for Disease Control and Prevention showed that the percentage of women over forty who had at least one mammogram rose from 54 percent in 1987 to 75 percent in 1990. Therapies are now available that were once unimaginable. Clot-busters, drugs used to unclog arteries during heart attacks, became standard treatment after they were approved for intravenous use in the mid-1980s. Even childhood vaccination programs are much improved. Within the last ten years, two vaccines have been added to the standard series. The hemophilus influenza B vaccine, given to protect infants against the most common cause of childhood meningitis, is given four times before age two. Its net cost is roughly $80 for the four shots. Another vaccine, against hepatitis B, is given three times by the age of six months. Its net cost is roughly $60. All of this costs money.

But a greater demand for useful services does not fully explain our predicament. In addition to growth in technology, medical costs are going up because of general inflation, population growth, and aging societies. These upward forces face every other industrial country, regardless of their delivery systems. Canada, Japan, and countries across Europe all have rising health-care costs.

Over the last decade, general inflation has accounted for roughly 40 percent of the rise in health-care costs, according to the Congressional Budget Office. The figure that is often cited to show how much faster medical costs have risen than general inflation is the consumer price index. From 1981 to 1991, medical prices rose more than twice as fast as the CPI. But the Congressional Budget Office, Congress's own accounting office, cautions against its facile use. Using the CPI as a measure of medical care has several problems. "A careful analysis shows that price measures are seriously flawed," the CBO warned, "because they do not adequately adjust for technological improvements." Better quality of care is not reflected in the CPI. The CPI is also is based on list price, not actual price. And fewer and fewer people are paying list price. A study of California hospitals in the 1980s found that list prices rose 70 percent but actual prices rose only 40 percent.

Another 10 percent of the rise in health-care costs over the past decade results from demographic changes. Since 1960, the U.S. population has grown between 1 and 2 percent a year. Not only are there more of us, we're older. Between 1950 and 1990, the segment of the population age sixty-five or older grew from 8 percent to more than 12 percent. Over the past decade, the percentage of the population that is eighty-five years old or older has tripled. And we are going to get even older. By the time that the entire baby-boom generation joins the ranks of the elderly, 20 percent of the population will be sixty-five or older. Our larger, older, and wealthier population demands more health care.

Although the onset of our chief complaint can be dated, much about it remains unexplained. Demographic trends are predictable. Inflation is measurable. Something else became the hallmark of rising costs. We were doing a poor job of mapping costs, of seeing where they would come from. It was like a disease with protean manifestations—you didn't quite know how it would progress. Efforts to control costs just seemed to aggravate them. Our technological and administrative efforts have worsened cost control—like some unforeseen complications of treatment.

Technological advances that held out the prospect of lowering costs by reducing hospital admissions failed to lower costs even though they did eliminate hospital time. Coronary angioplasty, in which a tiny catheter is threaded into blocked heart arteries, was meant to displace bypass surgery as the surgical procedure to open clogged, atherosclerotic blood vessels that supply the heart. Developed in the late 1970s, the new technique was far less invasive than open heart surgery, which required opening up the chest and putting the patient on a heart-lung bypass machine. Instead of a five-to-seven-day hospitalization, only an overnight stay for observation was needed.

But the new technology didn't save money by replacing the older operation. Instead, both procedures grew. By 1988, the number of angioplasties had risen to 227,000 from 26,000 in 1983, and the number of bypasses had also grown—from 191,000 in 1983 to 353,000 in 1988. By 1993, there would be an estimated 500,000 angioplasties.

Physician behavior partly explained the scenario. Angioplasties were lucrative for a different group of doctors than those who performed bypasses. Cardiologists, who rose from the rank of internists, did angioplasties, whereas thoracic surgeons did bypasses. Coronary arteries could now be unclogged by two groups of differently trained doctors. Invasive cardiologists, as those who do procedures such as angioplasty are called, earn considerably more than noninvasive cardiologists. In 1988, the median income for invasive cardiologists was $256,744, as opposed to $187,000 for noninvasive cardiologists, according to the Medical Group Management Association, a trade group.

But physician self-interest didn't account for the entire picture. The less grueling physical procedure meant that more people would be eligible, either because doctors thought they could tolerate the less invasive alternative or because patients were no longer afraid to undergo the procedure. In the case of angioplasty, older and sicker patients could tolerate it. As the population aged, more people developed heart disease amenable to surgical correction. And although the less invasive procedure was considerably cheaper than bypass, it often needed to be repeated, since blood vessels closed up after angioplasty in as many as one third of patients. And in order to do angioplasty, you needed to have surgical backup capable of doing bypass, just in case someone had a major blockage while undergoing angioplasty. (Even with more-minor procedures, you often need considerable backup, in case things don't go as planned.)

A similar story followed the introduction of another new technology, laparoscopic or minimally invasive surgery. Many operations that once required large incisions and long recuperative periods could now be performed by surgeons wielding small instruments inserted through a hollow tube. In some cases patients could even be discharged the day of surgery. Standard gallbladder surgery, which produces the type of long scar that President Lyndon Johnson once revealed to the American public, has been largely replaced by laparoscopic gallbladder removal. Instead of a six- to ten-inch scar, there are only several tiny cuts, and instead of a six-week recovery, most patients can return to work within a week. Generally, hospital stays have been cut from five days to twenty-four hours. Despite this, laparoscopic cholecystectomies, as the new procedures are known, haven't cut costs. At first, costs of the procedure went up. One Blue Cross/ Blue Shield medical director found that initially the average cost of the newer procedure was $7,523, compared to $6,013 for the older one—$1,510 more for an operation that then shaved 2.3 days off the length of hospitalization. But like many cost issues, this wasn't so straightforward. It wasn't just the incentives of fee-for-service medicine that rewarded doctors for doing more.

A later study of laparoscopic gallbladder removal at HMOs found that even though they had been able to drive the cost of the procedure down significantly, the HMOs were spending considerably more on gallbladder removals. The reason was that patients with mild symptoms who had resisted the open surgery, with its pain and lengthy recovery, now wanted to be cured. People had rationed their own care, not because of payment issues, but because of fear. New technology was removing that barrier to care.

Administrative efforts to lower costs also backfired. Insurers tried to cut hospital costs by decreasing and shortening admissions. Private insurers required subscribers to get second opinions prior to elective surgery. They also demanded preadmission authorization for nonemergency admissions and, in the case of emergency admissions, notice within forty-eight hours. Patients were often penalized if they didn't follow the rules, rules which they often forgot or didn't understand. One Polish maintenance worker at a major insurance company didn't speak English very well. After discharge from the hospital, where he had spent a few days to make sure that his chest pain wasn't a heart attack, he returned to work—only to show up at the employee health clinic wanting an explanation of the notice he had received from his insurer, which was also his employer. Since he hadn't notified them of admission within forty-eight hours of his emergency admission, they were denying a certain percentage of payment. That insurer acknowledged at internal meetings that they were unsure whether the preauthorization program was saving them any money, especially since they often reversed the denial, as they did with this man.

Set hospital fees have also been tried. The federal government, under Medicare, altered its method of payment. Using "diagnosis related groups" (known as DRGs), a payment scheme introduced in 1983, it paid hospitals a fixed price for treating each patient based on the diagnosis. No more unrestricted smorgasbord of fee-for-service care. The federal government now provides a lump-sum set price depending on the diagnosis. Hospitals make money if they treat a patient for less than what the DRG allows.

Insurers' efforts paid off in one sense. Hospital admissions dropped and the length of hospital stays decreased. But costs continued to climb. Between 1990 and 1991, hospital admissions dropped by 1.1 percent, according to the American Hospital Association. This was the largest drop in five years. The average length of stay was 5.3 days, the lowest ever. Despite the drop in admissions and in the length of stay, medical costs—including hospital costs—continued to soar. What had been unforeseen was the steep growth of outpatient hospital services. While inpatient costs slowed to 8 percent, outpatient costs were expected to grow 15 percent a year during the 1990s. Medical costs were very dynamic. Assuming that you were willing to let technological advances lead you, it was hard to predict where they would take you.

In the meantime, the drive to lower costs spawned an entirely new industry and created an administrative nightmare. A bureaucratic army arose, ready to battle the price hikes—all for their own fees. A whole industry, called utilization review, was created to make (their) profits by purportedly controlling costs (of others). As our costly and unwieldy system grew, it spawned a host of mini-industries that promised to rein in its excesses, to play David to the Goliath of health care. The health-care system was growing jobs endlessly, adding layer upon layer like a giant wedding cake. Actual patient care was becoming a smaller part of the picture, like remote figures viewed from an aerial photo.

Utilization review companies were one of the new players. UR firms promised to trim medical fat by shaving days off hospital admissions, by spotting claims that shouldn't be paid because of insurance terms, by denying or at least forestalling payments. The insurer (employer, government, or insurance company) could deny payment, either leaving patients to pick up the tab or providers to write it off. While only half of employers used utilization review in 1984, nearly all did by 1992.

The more than 350 utilization review companies that existed in 1992 had a dubious record overall. Looking at UR scrutiny of cataract operations under Medicare, the inspector general of the U.S. Health and Human Services Department found that in 1990 UR firms possibly eliminated $1.4 million in unnecessary cataract surgery, but at a cost of $13.3 million paid out to the UR industry. Large UR firms, like Intracorp in Berwin, Pennsylvania, were making nearly $300 million annually. By 1993, the rapidly growing cost-management industry was expected to generate $7 billion in revenue.

Utilization review only added to the health-care system's administrative costs, which at their current growth rate are expected to account for one third of health-care spending by 2003 and one half of health-care dollars by the year 2020. In 1987, we spent between $96.8 billion and $120.4 billion on administrative costs. This came to 19.3 to 24.1 percent of total health-care dollars that year. Between $400 and $497 per person was spent on administering health care rather than delivering it. While administrative costs rose 37 percent in real dollars between 1983 and 1987 in the United States, administrative costs actually fell in Canada. This difference in administrative costs accounts for roughly half of the difference in health-care spending between the two countries. The degree of waste in our complicated bureaucracy is phenomenal. Blue Cross/Blue Shield of Massachusetts, which insured 2.7 million subscribers in 1991, employed 6,682 people, more than it took to run Canada's entire system, then serving 25 million people.

If health-care upstarts turned the industry into a gimmicky

maze, the old guard did little to turn its advances into lower costs. The pharmaceutical industry is a prime example.

A congressional report found that pharmaceutical annual profit margins averaged 15.5 percent, more than triple the 4.6 percent profit margin of the average Fortune 500 company in the 1980s. In 1990, Merck and Syntex led the profits-as-percent-of-sales list, with 23.2 percent and 23.3 percent profit margins respectively.

The report, by the Senate's Special Committee on Aging, dismissed the pharmaceutical industry's claim that high profits and rapid inflation rates were needed to spur research and development. Using data supplied by the industry, the committee found that, in 1991, the drug industry planned to spend $1 billion more on marketing and advertising than it planned to spend on R & D—$10 billion compared with $9 billion.

The committee also cited the very high rate of inflation in costs of drugs that had long been on the market and were made by companies that showed little evidence of converting their profits to the development of new drugs. These drugs included:

- Tylenol with Codeine, a painkiller made by McNeil Pharmaceuticals that had been marketed since 1977, had a 16 percent annual inflation rate from 1985 to 1991. The company had not brought a new compound to market in the last five years.
- Synthroid, a thyroid supplement once made by Flint, has been available since 1938. Synthroid had a 15.5 percent yearly increase between 1985 and 1990. Flint brought no new compounds to market within the five-year period. (Flint, originally a division of Baxter, was bought by Boots in 1986.)
- Premarin, an estrogen replacement therapy used by postmenopausal women (a group that will grow as the baby-boom generation ages), has been on the market since 1956. On average, its price went up 21.5 percent yearly between 1985 and 1990—the highest rate listed in the report. Its price had increased every 8.5 months. Wyeth-Ayerst, its manufacturer, brought one new compound to market in five years. That one product was categorized by the Food and Drug Administration as having "little or no therapeutic gain over currently marketed drugs."
- Dilantin, used to control seizures, had been on the

market since 1953. Parke-Davis increased the drug's price over 11 percent annually, without bringing any new compounds to market over the previous five years.

The congressional report found that an increasing number of "new" drugs were in fact "me-too" drugs, drugs that merely duplicate others on the market and would hardly justify claims about high R & D costs. "Me-too" drugs also tend to require higher advertising budgets, since their intrinsic advantages don't sell the drug. When penicillin first hit the market, it didn't need much advertising—the drug worked.

Like many chief complaints, the illness often started long before the patient sought care. Like the patient with lactose intolerance whose gastrointestinal complaints had been going on for several years, something triggered him to complain, to seek care when he did. Maybe he just got health insurance, so he felt freer to seek medical care. Maybe a close friend developed cancer, and he suddenly worried that something was really wrong. If the problem didn't just start, a doctor wants to know why the patient is worried now.

Although Bill Clinton pushed health reform to center stage after he was elected president and appointed Hillary Rodham Clinton to head the health-reform task force, momentum already had been building for several years. Perhaps the reason lay in the complaints of those who were paying the bills. Most notably, the federal government.

For the first time, in 1991, the government spent more than households did in out-of-pocket health-care costs. The government was worried about what health care was doing to the national debt and what it would do to spending on other items. Our $312 billion annual deficit in 1992 was projected to soar to $514 billion in the year 2002, largely because of increased Medicare and Medicaid spending.

Health-care costs in 1991 consumed 20 percent of government revenues. The federal government's two major programs, Medicare and Medicaid, were growing by leaps and bounds. Run by the Health Care Financing Administration, an agency that had a budget of $230 billion by 1993, both programs were costing a lot more each year. But Medicaid, a joint federal-state program for the poor, was growing at a truly astonishing rate. It had grown 31 percent between 1990 and 1991, and 25 percent a year later. For neither Medicare nor Medicaid could the rise in costs be explained by the rise in number of people covered. For fiscal year 1992, Medicare was covering only 1.7 percent more people and Medicaid only 12 percent more.

Business was balking because it spent an increasing fraction of its costs on health care. Corporate health-care spending in 1992 was said to consume 45 percent of net corporate profits. General Motors estimated that it spent more on health care than on steel for each vehicle made. Chrysler, at $1,100 per vehicle, spent even more on health care than GM, at $929. On average, health-care costs added $1,086 to every car built in America. U.S. businesses complained that health-care costs were dulling their competitive edge. The Congressional Budget Office, however, disputed this argument, pointing out that businesses compensated for the increased costs by holding wages down.

Consumers also felt squeezed for a variety of reasons. Although most traditional health insurance policies still claimed 80 percent coverage, rising deductibles and limitations on coverage often reduced the effective coverage to 50 to 60 percent of the bill. Because employers paid more for health insurance instead of giving raises, real wages stagnated over the past two decades. And consumers paid higher payroll taxes to fund government health programs. Ultimately, as many economists point out, consumers always foot the bill—businesses, government, and insurance companies simply pass along their costs.

Because the poor tend to have inferior insurance and because health-care financing is regressive, poor households are especially strapped by medical costs. Based on the 1977 National Medical Care Expenditure Survey, the poorest 10 percent of households paid 14 percent of their income in out-of-pocket costs, whereas the wealthiest 10 percent of households paid 1.9 percent of their income for out-of-pocket costs. But even the middle class feels pinched. Nearly one fourth of people with private health insurance and one fifth of those with incomes greater than $50,000 were found to have deferred medical care because of financial concerns, according to a 1992 poll by Louis Harris. Medical costs have become the number-one cause of bankruptcy.

One reason that privately-insured consumers saw their costs rise was government cost-shifting. A study of hospital payments found that Medicare paid 88 percent of actual hospital costs, and Medicaid paid 82 percent, but private insurers paid 130 percent. In New Jersey, insured consumers picked up $900 million annually in hospital costs for the poor. Under a law called the

Uncompensated Care Trust Fund, a 19 percent surcharge was tacked onto the hospital bills of patients covered by union health plans and certain group health insurance plans. This additional revenue helped finance hospital care for roughly 800,000 uninsured New Jersey residents until a federal judge found the rate-setting scheme unenforceable. The law was deemed unenforceable not because of its blatant unfairness but because—as the unions argued—it forced them to pay for nonmembers' health care. The judge agreed that this was a violation of federal law. Violation of law or not, it was the wave of the future. Cost-shifting was the way costs were being cut. Governments, federal and state, shied away from raising taxes to cover the benefits they mandated. That would have been politically unpopular. Instead, they concealed the costs in consumers' pockets.

As we look at the major problem with health care—its cost—we can't lose sight of what part of the equation we can manipulate. Roughly half of the rise in spending has nothing to do with health care, but is due to general inflation and population shifts. The largest slice that could be varied—32 percent—comes from more frequent and more costly services, according to the Congressional Research Service. The remaining 17 percent comes from medical price inflation that exceeds general inflation. What this suggests is that cost containment must include pruning our use of high-tech care—something that people are often the least inclined to do. Fraud, waste, administrative costs, and physician salaries all contribute to rising costs. But saving big bucks means controlling technology.

CHAPTER 2

Access—More and More Are Losing It

Aᴄᴄᴇss ɪs ᴛʜᴇ ꜱᴇᴄᴏɴᴅ chief complaint. But until recently, one of the great differences between the problems of cost and access had been in the voices behind each complaint. Unlike the voices pushing for cost control, which represent some of the most powerful and best-organized forces in America, those crying for access are often weak and poorly organized.

In recent years, however, the middle class has increasingly had its access threatened, not by a shortage of medical facilities, but by the vagaries of health insurance. The result has been health-care angst. President Clinton's successful campaign slogan, "It's the economy, stupid," was paraphrased by Ronald Pollack, executive director of Families USA, a Washington-based consumer group that backed the administration's reform efforts. "It's peace of mind, stupid," he said, voicing the anguish of the insured and uninsured alike. His view could not have been better illustrated than by the case of James and Benny, two men who were sent to prison by federal prosecutors for fraud and conspiracy. Their crime had been switching identities to get health care.

James and Benny, friends from high school days, had been hiking in Tennessee when James fell off a thirty-foot cliff. Benny drove James, who was bleeding and unconscious, to the nearest emergency department, at Lewis County Community Hospital, according to a poignant account by Micki Siegel that appeared in *Good Housekeeping* magazine. Benny knew that James, a house-painter, was uninsured. Fearing they would be turned away, Benny gave James his identity, and with it his health insurance. James was transferred from the local emergency room to Maury

17

Regional and two days later to Vanderbilt University Medical Center because of the severity of his injuries. At Vanderbilt James underwent nine hours of surgery in the hope of preventing him from becoming paralyzed from the waist down. A neurosurgeon and orthopedist removed bony fragments and inserted steel rods.

Benny, a mechanic for Martin Marietta who was insured through the federal government, submitted the $41,000 medical bill. After the scheme was uncovered, he was summarily fired. Eight months later, in an early-morning raid, agents from the Federal Bureau of Investigation and the Drug Enforcement Administration, along with federal marshals and sheriff's deputies, stormed his house. After a jury trial, the judge sentenced Benny, his wife (because she had signed treatment authorizations), and James. He ordered Benny to repay the $41,000 tab—even though the hospitals reportedly had offered to write off the payment—and sentenced him to nine months in jail. His wife, a waitress, was sentenced to four months' house arrest for cooperating with the scheme. She was allowed, however, to go to work so that she could support their three young daughters, and she was permitted to visit her husband twice a month in jail. Of her $400 monthly income, the probation officer reportedly suggested that $300 go to repaying the hospital. James was sentenced to seven months in prison.

The government spent $350,000 to prosecute the case. (Ironically, a government report states that federal prosecutors rarely go after criminal health-care cases involving less than $100,000.) The prosecutor defended the decision to prosecute, claiming, according to newspaper reports, that the hospital would have treated James even without insurance, since there were anti-dumping laws that prohibited hospitals from refusing to treat deathly ill patients.

But most of us rightly wouldn't want to take that chance. While administering oxygen and intravenous fluids to an unconscious man would be considered life-saving (and thus illegal to withhold), transferring a stable patient to the best regional hospital for spinal surgery remains a more discretionary decision.

Had James, uninsured and denied care, become a paralyzed ward of the state, he could have regained access to the American health-care system. Self-employed and working, he would pay taxes toward Medicare and Medicaid but he was unable to afford his own health insurance. Unlike the CEO who earned $1 million a year and who got his health insurance tax-free, James, who took home $14,000 a year, would have had to buy his insurance with posttax dollars.

As happened in this case, access is generally viewed as an issue of being insured. Although that is the main determinant in the United States, it is not the only one. Access also involves issues of health policy and health-care delivery. Health reformers will neglect some of today's most serious problems if they assume that having insurance is synonymous with access. Access has to be judged in terms of the realistic ability to use needed services. If someone is insured but cannot afford the deductible, or if he belongs to an HMO that won't provide the services that he really needs, this person doesn't have adequate access. He is, however, insured. If he has to change doctors repeatedly because his insurance changes, he doesn't have good access.

As a matter of happenstance and not as a result of policy decisions, Americans have traditionally gotten health insurance through the workplace. The link occurred because of wage freezes during World War II, when employers competed for scarce workers by offering benefits instead of salary hikes.

But as insurance costs rose steeply—more than doubling between 1985 and 1991—many businesses couldn't afford to insure their workers. Even as employment grew by 15 million between 1980 and 1988, the number of privately insured Americans dropped by 5 million. More than half of those who had no medical insurance in 1990 were working. But by creating jobs without benefits (such as increasing overtime or hiring part-timers instead of full-time workers), the private sector could limit its liability. The burden of being uninsured but working fell disproportionately on the shoulders of employees already disadvantaged by job status—those who tended to be younger, less skilled, and lower paid.

But being insured through work is a fickle business. Even before the last recession really took hold, 63.6 million Americans were found in one study to lack health insurance for at least one month during a three-year period. The job-insurance link is like a revolving door, spewing Americans in and out of health insurance. A pink slip doesn't just mean unemployment—it also means no health insurance.

Government insurance through Medicaid (the insurance plan for the poor) isn't much more stable, since the levels of income eligibility can vary. In the early 1980s, eligibility for Medicaid was tightened—you had to be poorer to qualify. In 1992, many states

excluded children born before September 30, 1983, from their
Medicaid rosters if both parents worked, no matter how poor the
family. (Those born after 1983 were entitled to Medicaid benefits
until age eighteen, because the federal law had changed.) In 1992,
forty-five states imposed income eligibility for these children that
was set at 50 percent of poverty level. Modest changes in family
income could eliminate a child's health insurance.

Although the access problem has generally been defined by
citing the number of uninsured—nearly 39 million Americans in
1992—that mantralike number grossly understates the problem.
These are people who lack private insurance or government
insurance, such as Medicare and Medicaid. But in addition to the
uninsured, there are the "underinsured"—an estimated 20 million Americans whose health insurance is inadequate. They are
underinsured for any of several reasons: their deductibles are too
high relative to their income, their insurance excludes needed
preventive services or medical care for preexisting conditions,
their insurance is tied to a job that they will lose, their insurance
has a benefit cap that is lower than what they need. In the current
environment of soaring costs and fragmented efforts to control
them, the mushrooming caveats to health insurance mean that an
increasing proportion of insured would be more accurately classi-
fied as underinsured. Of insured working-age adults, 12 percent
said that illness caused major financial problems, according to a
1986 Robert Wood Johnson Foundation "Access to Health Care
Survey." If we add the uninsured and underinsured, we find
almost 60 million Americans do not have adequate health
insurance.

A striking feature of our "access" problem is the limited access
to appropriate care. But to address that issue brings up thorny
questions of what is appropriate care. Both uninsured and insured Americans can secure unlimited access to high-technology
care once they're moribund. Gasping for their last breath, both the
insured and the uninsured can probably gain access to a respirator in an intensive care unit. But in need of vaccinations or
treatment for an earache, they may have greater trouble.

Medicare, which pays a fortune for high-technology care, has
had a dismal record covering preventive services for the elderly.
Until 1993, Medicare did not pay for flu shots, though influenza is
a significant cause of illness and death in the elderly. A study of
Medicare spending found that 27.9 percent of Medicare funds
went to the 5.9 percent of Medicare enrollees who died within the

year. The Health Care Financing Administration, which oversees Medicare, found that reimbursements were consistently six times higher for patients who died during their hospital stay than for those who survived. The level of inappropriate "access" was even more disturbing because most people (70 percent in one study) say that they would decline life-sustaining treatment in the face of a poor prognosis. Not even those who get unlimited care seem to be getting what they want.

At the other end of the age spectrum, the access problem is even more disturbing. Children are often uninsured. In 1990, 8.4 million children had no health insurance at all—either private or public. (One source puts this figure much higher—12 million children with no health insurance and an additional 10 million who lack insurance for part of the year.) Forty percent of American children lacked employer-based medical insurance (the main type of health insurance for working-age Americans and their families) even though 85 percent lived in working families. Of 46 million children who had private health insurance that year, nearly 20 million were expected to be without coverage for some time by 1992. If the drop in employer-based coverage were to continue at the pace it had from 1977 to 1987 (and this was before the recession caused layoffs), it would have been expected that by the end of the century nearly half of all children would lack employer-based health insurance.

This loss of access to health insurance hit both low- and middle-income families, those with one or two wage earners, all races, rural and urban. It was worse if you were poor, but it was a trend that resonated throughout. No health planner could justify the fact that the money spent on the last six months of life for elderly patients under Medicare was roughly sixteen times the outlay of public funds on maternal and child-care programs.

Children also have skewed access to health care. Portia, a little girl who had no chance of meaningful brain function because she was born with most of her brain cocooned in a sac outside her skull, has been kept alive in a Washington rehabilitation hospital for over two years. She has required round-the-clock nursing since birth in 1991. Medicaid has paid more than half a million dollars so far. To make matters even worse, this child was born because the obstetrician refused the parents' request for an abortion when they were told of the child's prospects. The parents had been denied appropriate access to care.

Even with children, we let basic health care languish and use technology inappropriately. Although each dollar spent on vaccinations is said to save between $10 and $14 later, we let the immunization status of our children slide. If we compare the number of one-year-olds in the United States who are fully immunized against polio with rates around the world, we find we rank behind Bulgaria, North Korea, and Albania, according to 1992 data from Unicef. In 1991, pertussis cases were double the number in 1981, rubella cases were five times the number in 1988, and the country was in the third year of a measles epidemic. Although there were fewer than 1,500 cases of measles by 1983, there were more than 27,000 in 1990.

The problem isn't limited to uninsured children. Among those who are privately insured, nearly one half of employer-based insurance policies and almost two thirds of preferred-provider organizations exclude routine vaccinations, such as those that wiped out polio and diphtheria. Increasingly, even insured children use already overburdened public clinics for immunizations. Physicians in Dallas reported almost a sevenfold increase in children referred to public clinics for immunization from 1979 to 1988.

Problems faced by those children covered by Medicaid highlight why insurance and access aren't synonymous. A 1991 review of the measles epidemic by the Centers for Disease Control and Prevention found that 75 percent of preschool measles cases in New York were among children entitled to Medicaid; in Milwaukee it was 86 percent.

Medicaid fee schedules are often so low that children are only semi-insured. Rates and policies vary by state, because the program is determined and funded at both the state and federal levels, but a glimpse at one state's reimbursement rates offers a look at the problem. Leafing through New York State's April 1993 fee schedule, a 437-page manual, showed that the state allowed a maximum fee of $6.50 for an initial hospital visit by a primary care doctor. Office fees were slightly higher—$7.50. Laboratory fees took the absurdity one step further. For a urinalysis, used to diagnose problems like urinary infections, Medicaid allowed 50 cents. For a blood test used to establish anemia, Medicaid paid 80 cents. Providers were also faced with the hassle of trying to collect.

Medicaid's vaccine policy shows a glaring disregard for real economic factors. Several states reimbursed physicians for administering childhood immunizations at less than the cost of the vaccine. Seventeen states refused payment for follow-up visits when more than one office visit was required to complete an immunization series.

As a result of the grossly inadequate fee schedule for childhood immunizations, an increasing number of children aren't cared for by private pediatricians—even those who accept Medicaid—but are sent to already overcrowded public health facilities. A working mother or one who has to pick up another child from school may not have hours to wait in a clinic. The "hurry-up-and-wait" approach lowers access by raising the level of frustration to unbearable heights.

Parents who fail to immunize their children are sometimes punished. Maryland, for instance, proposed reducing Aid to Families with Dependent Children benefits for families that failed to immunize their children. Under Medicaid, however, Maryland allowed only $73.33 for immunizing a child at fifteen months, even though the usual and customary charges were calculated to be $125. The fee was far too low to secure care by most community physicians. And if the child was found unable to be vaccinated at that visit, which could easily happen if the child was sick or unable to tolerate four vaccines at once, Maryland allowed no payment for a follow-up visit.

A pilot program in Philadelphia that enrolled Medicaid patients in HMOs also showed that the details of health-care delivery—not just insurance status—determine true access. Many parents who were enrolled in the program didn't keep appointments for their children and thus failed to get them immunized. One reason turned out to be that some doctors wouldn't schedule more than two children at one visit. If parents had more children, they needed multiple visits. Parents with many children couldn't play by these rules.

If access to care needs to be looked at in terms of appropriateness of care and the realities of delivery systems, one of the new issues will be continuity of care under managed care. Patients can easily lose their doctor if they change plans or if a plan changes its rules. They may find that they can keep their gynecologist or pediatrician, but not both, because each doctor belongs to a different plan. But long-standing doctor-patient relationships are crucial. They foster trust and offer a diagnostic edge. Understanding a patient's psyche—like knowing whether he tends to be stoic or depressive—and knowing how an illness has played itself out over time, offer the doctor an enormous advantage. A written medical record—no matter how detailed—can never substitute.

When managed-care plans change rules in midstream—as they often do—patients may find their access jeopardized. As the following New York examples show, doctors may leave plans or be barred from continuing certain services. PruCare, Prudential's HMO-without-walls, planned to change its reimbursement policy. Instead of paying fee-for-service as they had done, they announced they were switching to a captitation system—doctors would get a low monthly retainer for having a patient on their panel whether the patient never showed up or showed up frequently. More doctors balked than PruCare predicted. The company scuttled its plan for converting to capitation by November 1, 1993, and put it off until January 1994. How an HMO pays and treats its doctors affects who will be working there.

Another New York HMO-without-walls, Oxford, also made a decision that affected patient care. In 1993, Oxford decided that certain specialists who were now joining their network of doctors could practice only their specialty: they couldn't be general internists for Oxford patients as well. When an oncologist who enjoyed both his general and specialty practice balked, he was told that was company policy. In this and similar cases, patients may find that their HMO has limited their access to many highly trained doctors who like to provide primary-care medicine as well as practice their specialty.

Reformers may be promising blanket access to clearly defined benefits, but it is only the fine print that determines the realities. And that fine print changes. The discontinuity of care that existed when health insurance was linked to the workplace could be duplicated by linking providers to managed-care plans.

The problems of access differ, mainly according to patient income. The poor are victims of the discrepancy between insurance and access because Medicaid's fee structure is so low that it doesn't allow them to use mainstream health care.

For the middle class, access and insurance were largely synonymous until deductibles started to rise and insurance companies excluded a growing number of people.

Managed care may solve these problems of access—but not without creating others. Choice will be bartered for security.

CHAPTER 3

Insurance—Now You See It, Now You Don't

A YOUNG MARRIED COUPLE both had health insurance, each through work. When she had trouble getting pregnant, she tried to switch to her husband's policy because it turned out that his plan—not hers—covered infertility. His insurance plan declined: her infertility was a preexisting condition. A short time later, she discovered that without any high-tech medical assistance she had become pregnant. She again tried to switch plans, having realized that her husband's larger employer was able to offer more generous benefits. His plan again refused, now because she had another preexisting condition: pregnancy. After she delivered prematurely by emergency cesarean section, it turned out her health insurance wasn't going to pay 80 percent of the bill as she had assumed. It was going to deduct 10 percent of whatever it would have normally paid. That wasn't because she hadn't met her deductible. It was because she had failed to notify her plan within forty-eight hours of admission. Distracted by an emergency C-section and not having looked at her insurance plan for five years, she simply forgot to call.

For many Americans, the system of health insurance has faded into chaos. It blends a bureaucracy's compassion with Kafkaesque logic. In 1992, there were more than 1,500 insurers (including 1,150 commercial carriers, 73 nonprofit Blue Cross/Blue Shield plans, and 569 HMOs). Each had its own underwriting principles. Companies view the same risks differently, so that high blood pressure might mean paying higher premiums or it might mean having the condition excluded from coverage. Health plans fall under different regulatory jurisdictions. Insurance plans are

25

regulated by state insurance laws, and all fifty states have individual rules. Self-insured plans escape state regulations and fall under federal law instead. And insurance companies write differing policies tailored to each employee group. One New York doctor received a package from a major HMO, detailing more than sixteen different managed-care plans that it had for employers in his area. Some plans included infertility services, some didn't. Copayments varied. Some were self-insured, others were backed by the insurer. But each plan—bearing the same HMO name— was unique.

Only Medicare, the federal insurance plan for the elderly, protects its beneficiaries with the security and consistency that should characterize health insurance. Whereas only 1 percent of the elderly were uninsured in 1992, 17 percent of those under age sixty-five lacked health coverage. The federal government has also interceded to protect Medicare recipients from being duped by insurance plans they don't understand by streamlining Medigap policies, which were designed to supplement Medicare coverage. In 1992, the federal government prohibited companies from selling more than ten plans, each with standardized benefits that don't overlap existing Medicare coverage. The move forced insurers to abandon their dizzying array of useless policies. Unfortunately for the elderly, similarly worthless policies are cropping up in the nursing home market. But the rest of us wade through a morass of insurance practices.

Tax policies that benefit both employees and employers have cemented the link between employment and health insurance. While payroll taxes take an increasing bite out of wages, health premiums are paid with pretax dollars. A $1,000 increase in health benefits is worth more than $1,000 increase in wages because benefits—unlike wages—aren't taxed. While policies with lower deductibles are more expensive than those with high deductibles, a comparison shopper might choose to buy such a plan because of the tax law. If the premium is paid for with pretax dollars it may be cheaper to buy the expensive policy rather than pay high deductible out-of-pocket costs with posttax dollars. Many people don't want to relinquish this system.

Employers (assuming that they are incorporated businesses) deduct 100 percent of premiums as a business expense. Unlike wages, they don't pay payroll taxes on this money. This amounts to a $50 billion federal tax subsidy to employers. The favorable tax treatment of insurance premiums, which grows as premiums rise, means higher taxes for some, lower services for others, and a higher deficit for us all. Thus tax law favors buying health insurance plans with low deductibles. The 1945 McCarran-Ferguson Act, which allowed insurance companies to share data with each other without violating antitrust laws, reinforces the sense that the insurance industry grew under the protective wing of government.

In general, people who work for large companies have fared better than those who work for small companies. Individuals who buy insurance on their own have fared the worst. But members of every group have run into problems. And many people have found themselves being tossed from one group into the uncertainty of another. Retirees, who thought their benefits secure, have become uninsured long before they qualify for Medicare at age sixty-five. But, before looking at how policyholders have really fared, it's worth looking at the general behavior of the insurance industry.

Over the years, an increasing number of Americans have found that they can't afford health insurance, that insurance companies don't want to sell them policies, or that when they file a claim, it is at least partly denied. Difficulties cut across all insurers, to greater or lesser degrees. But as health insurers now reinvent themselves as the compassionate, rational deliverers of managed care, we should remember their past. Rather than band together to solve the problem of escalating costs, insurers sought to exclude the sick and the potentially sick.

Curious in today's discussion of health reform is that many proposals actually give the health insurance industry more clout than it previously had. Given its track record of power devoid of ethical obligation—which it justified by claiming to hold costs down for the people it didn't exclude—placing further trust in the insurance industry is a strange move. These are the same companies that once opposed payment for preventive health services. Now they encourage them. Vaccines and screening tests were once denied because they were considered health-related rather than illness-related. Some people even argued that they shouldn't be covered because preventive services increase the cost of health insurance. Giving this industry more control is a bit like having the fox guard the henhouse.

If you were a doctor listening to a patient describe a chronic disease, you would consider a history of their disease highly relevant to deciding on treatment. If a patient had asthma for fifteen years, but had only occasional mild symptoms, you would give him an asthma medication, known as a bronchodilator, to take periodically when needed. But if a patient complained of daily severe attacks, you would put him on inhaled steroids continuously. Two very different strategies based on history— even if their symptoms were identical the day they walked in your office.

Yet health-care reformers seem willing to turn their backs on the history of the insurance industry. Recast as managed care, insurers are expected to operate with different standards. The problem is that the industry is—by its own admission—in business purely to make money. The industry never had a social mandate.

But insurers developed a lot of power. Given the clout insurers exert on how medicine is practiced, there developed a gaping cleft between the power behind health care and responsibility for its outcomes. What insurers paid for is what the public got. Without reimbursement, new procedures are either dead in the water or applied on a limited basis. While the industry's grip on medical practice usually focuses on the diffusion of technology (e.g., there will be more MRIs if insurance pays for them), insurers have had profound effects on the types of treatment offered.

Reimbursement rates allowed fees for procedures to soar, unhindered by market constraints. At the same time, until their reincarnation as managed-care providers, insurers refused payment for vaccinations and screening tests, such as Pap smears. And they showed little innovation or flexibility in covering new services, for fear that doing so would simply pave the way for more financial liability on their part.

They avoided paying for "lifestyle" therapies, even when medically preferable. One insurer that I worked for declined to pay for weight-reduction programs for obese diabetics, even though weight loss can be curative whereas drugs are only palliative. Company officials were very reluctant to wedge open a door that was securely shut. They admitted that they feared it would permit other, nondiabetic policyholders to demand that their weight reduction efforts be subsidized. Rather than write appropriate guidelines for payment, it was safer to enforce a blanket denial. The officials acknowledged that weight reduction was the treatment of choice for an overweight diabetic. They couldn't even use medical ignorance to defend their position.

A study by a Dartmouth professor of community and family

medicine found that phone consultations improved care and cut costs in the management of chronic disease, a finding in accord with what many primary care doctors already suspected. But phone consultations have never been reimbursed by insurers. The federal government's Office of Technology Assessment found that involving physicians was "crucial" for providing high-quality care when patients were treated with home infusion for diseases such as cancer, AIDS, or other serious infections requiring intravenous antibiotics. But despite these findings, Medicare does not pay doctors to oversee home-care patients. Insurers, both private and government, have resisted paying for broader services—particularly ones that doctors traditionally provide for free.

The history of private health insurance in America should sound a cautionary note. Rather than doing what insurance is intended to do, namely, pool or distribute risk, health insurers choose to try to eliminate risk. In other words, they try to cast out the sick and minister to the well. Americans have been carved into insurance niches. Increasingly, they fall between the cracks.

Insurers have devoted increasing time and money to weeding out the bad risks, since they found that 70 percent of all medical expenses were incurred by 10 percent of the population. The percentage of policies that have some exclusion or surcharge for higher-than-normal risk has risen steadily through the years. Where exclusions once focused on life-threatening, serious illnesses, they have grown to include common maladies such as migraine headaches, arthritis, hemorrhoids, varicose veins, and allergies.

Ferreting out the bad risks isn't cheap. Of $157.8 billion in premium revenues in 1987, $18.7 billion went to overhead and profits. Overhead expenses consumed 11.9 percent of premium revenues, compared with 3.2 percent in public insurance programs, such as Medicare and Medicaid (although these low figures omit some overhead costs that have been shifted onto providers, regional insurance companies, and local governments).

Some administrative costs are due to corporate largess. Pennsylvania Insurance Department officials found that executives of Blue Cross plans in its home state had spent $50,000 on a conference table, more than $234,000 on sporting events over four years, and $53,000 on club memberships in one year. But much of the cost comes from trying to minimize risks or avoid claims payments. Underwriting (the process of calculating someone's

risk), documenting eligibility, calculating deductibles, and deciding which services are covered benefits is very costly. Private
insurers' administrative costs rose nearly 300 percent between
1980 and 1990, whereas benefits rose less than 200 percent. As the
system grew more costly and unwieldy, costs were passed on to
consumers. Unlike businesses that suffer when they become
inefficient, insurance companies simply pass along their costs.

A surge in medical testing has enabled insurers to delve deeper
into the health status of applicants—evaluating their chances of
developing a disease rather than merely having it. Whereas
insurers once looked at cardiograms to see whether someone had
a heart attack, they now also check serum cholesterol levels to see
whether someone is at increased risk of developing one. Genetic
testing allows insurers a crystal ball with which to peer into the
future, segregating those at high risk, also known as the
"asymptomatic ill." Amniocentesis, which allows genetic testing
in utero, could mean that a child enters the world uninsurable,
the insurance industry's equivalent of India's untouchables. Even
if insurers don't order a test, they usually obtain complete access
to medical records, allowing them to use information that isn't
even relevant to the disease in question.

Insurers don't hesitate to defend their positions using spurious
arguments when they seek to avoid paying claims. The same
company that denied payment for weight reduction that could
cure diabetes refused to reimburse patients for in vitro fertilization because it didn't "cure" infertility. They weren't the only
company to argue their positions on shaky medical ground. In
1978, for example, the Travelers Insurance Company fought a suit
by one of its policyholders to be reimbursed for Laetrile and
nutritional therapy. The man had received the worthless treatment after having had part of his cancerous right lung surgically
removed. Travelers defended its position, not by saying that the
alternative treatment was unproven, but by claiming that the man
was not sick within the policy's definition because his cancer had
been removed through surgery. Anyone with an iota of knowledge of lung cancer would know that the cancer couldn't possibly
be considered cured as soon as it was scooped out. Since one
could safely assume that any insurance company would know
this, one could only presume that this was an attempt at legal
legerdemain and not an act of concerned good faith.

Sometimes insurance companies refuse payment, saying that
the previous payments have been made in error. They effectively

change their minds in midstream. One man, after undergoing cardiac rehabilitation for nine months and having thirty-seven claims paid, received a request for a $6,512.77 refund from his insurer. Although this insurer covered cardiac rehabilitation, the company claimed that this man did not fit their guidelines because of his prerehabilitation profile. Although they allowed him to incur these charges, paying his claims and never notifying him of a possible difficulty, they felt he was responsible. The insurer put an internal lien on his policy, refusing to pay any other medical claims until he returned the money. Following a complaint to the New York Insurance Department, the insurer rescinded its refund request and removed the lien.

The insurance industry has operated under a shroud of secrecy that it claims is needed to prevent abuses and safeguard companies' competitive edges. Companies claim that they will draw high-risk patients if they let potential customers know that they cover a certain disease without restriction or liberally pay for "experimental" treatments. The potential for adverse selection is the reason for keeping policyholders in the dark. A buyer's efforts to find out what a company will pay for and what another one won't are rebuffed. As a result, in today's market, a person cannot comparison-shop, except in such a schematic way that the effort may prove useless.

But insurance secrets, revealed only in adversity, can spell disaster. Sometimes policies are clear but not divulged. One couple, while waiting to adopt a child, approached their insurance agent to buy a policy that would automatically add the child to the parents' policy. Assured that this prominent nationwide insurer would do so, they bought a policy. Several months later, they became the delighted parents of an infant, healthy apart from a heart murmur of questionable significance. Like almost all new parents, they wouldn't have considered turning down their child.

The agent wrote a letter to confirm that the baby had been added to the parents' policy, and the parents paid the additional premium for the child. Six weeks later, without warning, a letter arrived. It had been a mistake. The insurer had refused to add the infant. A spokesman for the Health Insurance Association of America, the insurance industry's Washington-based trade group, confirmed that various insurers handled adopted children differently, but he could not reveal which company had told him what. Some companies would have added any child within the first thirty days of arrival in the new home, other companies would apply their regular underwriting criteria for any child older than thirty days.

There are many other ways to get tripped up. While the standard indemnity policy may promise 80 percent payment, not all 80 percents are equal. An insurer might pay 80 percent, but of "usual and customary fees" in your geographic area. A consumer might assume that these fees are standard. But while some insurers set these fees at the ninetieth percentile, others used the fiftieth percentile as the maximum they would allow. For instance, a patient with a $2,000 tab would be reimbursed $1,600 under a policy that regarded the total cost as reasonable and customary, but only $800 under a policy that allowed $1,000 for the treatment. Until he was reimbursed, the patient wouldn't know whether his out-of-pocket expenses would be $400 or $1,200. He pays his nickel and takes his chances, since he certainly never got a brochure from the insurance company that explained these subtleties in bold print.

Some insurers cap specific fees. A major New York insurer selling indemnity policies in the late 1980s issued one that promised 80 percent payment of charges for a semiprivate hospital room. But Mutual of New York, which no longer sells such policies, capped the hospital charge at $400 a day. With hospital beds being charged then at a daily rate of $650, that left patients liable for $330 a day in non-covered room and board charges, even though they thought they had standard 80 percent coverage.

Policyholders may run into problems in ways that even the wary among us would never have considered. Insurers have the right to sell policies to other insurers. In 1993, the ITT Hartford Life Insurance Companies announced that they intended to transfer $820 million of group medical and dental plans to the Massachusetts Mutual Life Insurance Company. Although the terms of the insurance policy cannot be changed, time spent choosing an insurance company based on its financial stability or record for paying claims could be totally wasted. Consumers can refuse the transfer, but generally insurers are under no obligation to inform policyholders of their intent to transfer or of the consumer's right to refuse.

Many companies, including Mutual of New York, the ITT Hartford Life Insurance Company, and Aetna, engaged in the practice, known colloquially as "policy transfer" and in insurance argot as "assumption reinsurance." In 1991, when Aetna dropped their individual health insurance business, it sold 108,000 policies to Mutual of Omaha. The letter that Aetna sent its policyholders omitted the fact that policyholders could refuse. Although states generally allow policy owners to refuse a transfer, states impose markedly different rules on a company's obligation to notify people of this right. Writing a check to the new company or not responding to the notice of transfer is often seen as a legal consent. Although these transfers may look like banks selling mortgages, there is a vast difference. In the bank scenario, the consumer has already received the service. In the insurance one, the consumer is paying for a service not yet received—and one that, if it is not available when needed, can financially ruin him. At the end of 1993, the National Association of Insurance Commissioners adopted model legislation requiring that policyholders be notified and be able to refuse the transfer. But each state will have to turn this into law.

While policy transfer is certainly a hidden potential problem, the most threatening behind-the-scenes liability for patients is the variation in policies that comes from medical judgment calls. Standardized benefits are just not standardized at the cutting edge of medicine. They simply change too quickly. Most policies, including the Health Security Plan presented to Congress by the Clinton task force in its educational session called "health-care university," exclude experimental treatment. Benefits not covered by the Health Security Plan included "Investigational Treatments (except for Medically Necessary or Appropriate Care provided as part of an Approved Research Trial)." But cancer treatment often involves investigational treatment not given as part of a research trial, usually referred to as "off-label" use of drugs. For instance, Taxol, a drug that was approved for ovarian cancer, was used by many cancer experts because it had shown significant promise for advanced breast cancer—even though it had not been approved by the Food and Drug Administration for that use. Fortunately, most oncologists know from following developments in their field that certain drugs have shown promise before the FDA actually approves them for that use.

Insurers generally have not taken the lead in trying to resolve the problem by backing clinical trials that aim to test the effectiveness of new treatments. Instead, patients have often been forced to incur large bills and then sue for reimbursement. In 1991, Blue Cross/Blue Shield headquarters suggested to its member insurance companies that they consider paying part of the costs of bone marrow transplants for women with advanced breast cancer, but only after Blue Cross had already been sued by patients. What patients don't know is that there is a lot of variation from one insurance plan to another. "The company that does the best in paying for clinical trials is Aetna. MetLife is close behind," said Grace Powers Monaco, formerly the public member of the Food and Drug Administration's oncological drug advisory committee. A lawyer whose daughter died of cancer, she has advised both insurers and patients. Monaco added that "Aetna will also pay for you on or off trial as long as you match the clinical protocol," meaning that patients can be treated by their own oncologist rather than switch to one who is formally participating in the study.

That insurers refuse to pay for "experimental" but mainstream cancer treatment has long been a significant problem. It highlights the pitfalls of businessmen, not clinicians, setting clinical policies—especially in fields that are changing rapidly. According to a report by the government's General Accounting Office, one third of all drug therapy of cancer treatment involves off-label use of drugs. The GAO found that 62 percent of the oncologists in their survey were hospitalizing chemotherapy patients—rather than treating them on an outpatient basis—solely to ensure that patients would be reimbursed for treatment, since insurers were less restrictive about hospital treatment. The GAO also found that two thirds of the cancer specialists surveyed "reported 'moderate' to 'very great' difficulties staying abreast of shifts in reimbursement policy." The insurers named as giving them the most difficulty—requiring them to actually abandon their preferred treatment—were those who administer Medicare in each state.

The most vulnerable people in today's insurance market are individuals who buy their own insurance rather than getting it through work and employees of small groups. Since individuals account for only 10 to 15 percent of the insured population, they generally don't get as much attention as those employed in small businesses. But this has been a very fragile sector. Of more than 2 million new individual policies written each year, nearly one fifth had exclusions, higher-than-standard premiums, or both, according to a 1987 survey by the Office of Technology Assessment, the research arm of Congress. Eight percent of individual applicants were deemed uninsurable. Some of those were uninsurable not because of ill health but because of occupational or financial reasons or place of residence. Three insurers reported to OTA that they had used indirect methods, such as interviewing the applicant's neighbors, to determine whether a male applicant was homosexual, trying to ferret out a risk for AIDS. In their efforts to exclude any high-risk person, the fifty then-largest HMOs denied membership to one fourth of individual applicants.

Entire small businesses can find themselves viewed as unacceptable risks. Employees of beauty shops, physicians' offices, hotels, restaurants, and trucking firms are "redlined"—the insurance term for being unwanted. They are targeted because insurers find them to be high users of medical services. Just how many people fail to secure standard insurance policies (policies without premium hikes or waivers) offers a look at how many people are at risk of inadequate insurance or no insurance at all.

Theoretically, higher premiums in the individual and small-group market reflect higher risks due to the small base over which to spread the risk. Certainly, administrative costs are higher, accounting for 40 percent of the cost of premiums in businesses with one to four employees. But since large groups have the clout to force discounts from providers, individuals and small groups also see their own costs rise simply because of cost-shifting. Their premiums rise to reflect a greater risk that has to do with employment rather than health. Some of the "efficiencies" achieved by large employers or government are, in reality, cost-shifting.

Individual applicants and members of small groups are vulnerable, not just because of their higher insurance costs, but because underwriting, the process of assessing an individual's medical risk, can make them uninsurable. Certain states, including New York, ended the practice by mandating community rating, in which all applicants in one geographic area are charged the same, regardless of age, sex, or medical history.

Small-business owners have an increasingly tough time finding affordable, usable insurance. Since the percentage of the work force in this sector has grown, both because job growth has occurred in this sector and because the insurance industry expanded its definition of "small group," those with employer-based health insurance working for small firms increasingly find themselves in a more vulnerable market. Whereas small groups used to be defined as between three and twenty-five employees, fifty to one hundred employees is no longer uncommon.

A look at the percentage of uninsured working for small businesses shows how threatened the small-business sector has become. While 87 to 99 percent of large firms were able to offer health insurance in 1990, only 26 percent of firms with fewer than twenty-five workers were able to do so. Looking at the phenomenon from another angle showed that among companies not offering health insurance, 98 percent had fewer than twenty-five workers. Half of all uninsured employees work in small businesses. It isn't that small businesses are less concerned about employees, it is that they have fewer options. Many find that when they do buy insurance, sudden and steep premium hikes force them to drop coverage—especially when insurers use artificially low initial rates to recruit new business. These low rates tend to fade quickly once the exclusion of preexisting conditions expires. Once workers are eligible to file claims, the insurer prices their premiums out of reach. The practice is sufficiently widespread to have a name: churning. Companies have to switch insurers when they can't afford to renew. Only if state insurance laws protect consumers will small-group members not be subject to the exclusion, once again, of their preexisting conditions.

Although individuals and small group members are the most vulnerable, those who work for large companies can be trapped in the loopholes of self-insurance. Trying to stem rising medical costs, a growing number of companies have become self-insured rather than purchase policies from insurance companies. Their plans are regulated by federal legislation rather than state insurance law.

When Congress passed the Employee Retirement Income Security Act (ERISA) in 1974, however, only 5 percent of the work force was covered by self-insured plans. ERISA was mainly designed to protect pension plans rather than lay the foundation for health benefits. In the past, only large firms would self-insure, but now small and medium companies are following the trend. A 1991 study by A. Foster Higgins, the benefits consulting firm, found that 22 percent of companies with fewer than one hundred employees were self-insured—compared with only 8 percent in 1988. By 1992, almost two thirds of U.S. employers were self-insured, according to a survey of 2,000 mainly large employers by A. Foster Higgins. Roughly 71 million American workers had health benefits under ERISA rather than being covered by true medical insurance.

Self-insured companies reap several advantages. They are exempt from state insurance mandates, which vary widely from state to state but can require coverage of many more services than a self-insured plan might be inclined to offer. Some states require treatment of alcoholism, coverage of acupuncture for pain, payment for in vitro fertilization, maternity benefits. Self-insured plans escape these expensive constraints.

Since self-insured plans aren't insurance companies, they also avoid state taxes (usually 2 to 3 percent) on premiums that private insurance companies and some of the Blue Cross/Blue Shield plans pay. Self-insured companies also retain the use of the capital that would otherwise have gone to the insurers.

While commonly called "health insurance," these plans are not—they are "employee benefit plans." Technically, they aren't insurance plans because they don't transfer risk from one entity to another. The result is that employees "insured" under ERISA lack the protection that state laws provide for those who hold policies from insurance companies. To most users, there is no perceptible difference. To some employees, the difference has meant disaster.

The case that drew national attention to the vulnerability of those with health benefits rather than insurance was that of John McGann. An employee of H & H Music Company in Houston since 1982, McGann developed AIDS in 1987. After he started to file insurance claims, the company chose to become self-insured, dropping its group health insurance. H & H Music then slapped a $5,000 lifetime cap on AIDS treatment, a cap that is absurdly low for any major illness. H & H's $1 million lifetime cap for medical treatment had been amended for one case and one illness. The legality of this maneuver was upheld by the U.S. Court of Appeals for the Fifth Circuit. The U.S. Supreme Court, at the urging of the Justice Department, refused to hear the appeal.

The appellate court ruled that under ERISA, employers had "an absolute right to alter the terms of medical coverage available to plan beneficiaries." ERISA, the federal legislation designed to standardize employee pension and medical plans, preempts state laws.

Even if the McGann case were the only one of its kind—which it isn't—it deserves all the attention it can get. While the tampering with coverage was appalling on humanitarian grounds, it is a very specific reminder that health insurance without regulation is no health insurance at all. AIDS was the disease singled out in McGann's case—but any and all diseases could be substituted. The potential is unlimited. Employers could slash their costs by imposing low caps on Alzheimer's, cancer, alcoholism, diabetes, multiple sclerosis. It makes a mockery of health insurance: It insures you—unless, of course, you need it.

Other groups of Americans are also burned by the health insurance chaos. Many who cannot find policies are forced to take refuge in what turn out to be fraudulent schemes. In 1989, 5,000 people were left stranded with a total of $1.9 million in unpaid claims when their "insurance company," Cap Staffing Inc. of Charlotte, North Carolina, went belly-up. The insurer was technically a "multiple employer welfare association," a group that aims to pool small businesses in order to purchase health insurance as a larger entity. But many MEWAs turned out to be pyramid schemes. In 1991, six men were indicted on charges of federal fraud in the Cap Staffing affair. In another scheme, the federal government charged the International Forum of Florida Health Benefit Trust with defrauding 43,000 people of $29 million in premiums.

At least 400,000 Americans fell victim to such health plans between 1988 and 1990, the General Accounting Office estimated, leaving many of those who had developed serious illnesses bankrupt and unable to purchase real health insurance. Like the self-insured plans, MEWAs also escape regulation at the state level.

Another group victimized by the shifting of insurance status comprises retirees, roughly 13 million of whom receive health benefits from their former employers. They have been hard hit when companies decide to curtail or rescind their promises of health-care benefits in the golden years. Not only are older people more likely to need health insurance, but they may be financially vulnerable, trying to live on fixed incomes or pensions. Companies, having promised to pay retiree health costs when health costs were a shadow of their current rates, may have bitten off more than they can or want to chew. Analysts say that U.S. businesses carry a $98 billion to $145 billion liability for the health costs of employees who retired by 1988. If you add in the potential cost of those workers who were still working in 1988, the liability is more than double.

Companies, trying to curtail costs and to comply with accounting rules set by the Financial Accounting Standards Board that require them to set aside funds to cover benefits promised to retirees, have added escape clauses which allow them to change or cut benefits at will. The 1990 FASB rule 106 caused companies to cast retired employees into a health insurance void. As Uwe Reinhart, a political economist who has been active in the debate on health-care reform, put it, "That strategy will help hitherto deceived shareholders, but its victims will be unsophisticated retired American workers who probably could not have known better." What were thought of as lifetime benefits can come to a screeching halt long before Medicare kicks in. DuPont, Caterpillar, Unisys, and McDonnell Douglas are among the large corporations that recently cut retiree health benefits.

In one of the ironies of our health insurance system, more insurance can increase rather than minimize your risk. Some families that have two insured breadwinners have found that two health insurance policies can make matters worse. This conundrum is made possible by companies feuding over who will pay. The rules have grown so complex that even the insurers can find it difficult to sort out.

Insurance plans generally coordinate benefits, meaning that when a patient files a claim, the insurer checks what benefits the person might be entitled to under any other plan. Most plans now carry "nonduplication of benefits" clauses, meaning that if both plans pay 80 percent of claims, they cannot be combined to pay more than 100 percent.

But what insurers call "coordination of benefits" is sometimes more aptly called "claims hot potato." While children used to be covered under their fathers' plans (known as the "gender rule"), this practice is no longer automatic. Instead, many companies attach the children to the policy held by the parent whose birthday falls earlier in the year. When one company uses the "gender rule" and the other uses the "birthday rule," the result can be disastrous. Nearly four years after the birth of a premature baby, only $3,840 of a $344,000 hospital bill had been paid, because each parent's employer (both of which were self-insured) said the other plan was liable. The gender-rule policy and the birthday-rule policy had canceled each other out.

It would be wrong, however, to infer from this that having one policy is safer. Working parents have been left in the lurch by "phantom" coordination of benefits. An employee's plan may insist on coordinating benefits with those that the other spouse might have had, had the second spouse opted to maintain his or her company's plan. The fact that there is no other policy is considered irrelevant. Unlike the parents with the premature baby who were worse off because they had two policies, these parents would be worse off because they had only one.

Although Medicare has worked well to protect its beneficiaries, it would be wrong to conclude that public insurance is automatically more straightforward. Medicaid, the joint federal and state insurance program for the poor, has numbed many minds. New York State provided a 135-page manual to physicians that was the instruction booklet for completing a 1-page bill. South Carolina once required pregnant women to complete a 43-page questionnaire when applying for Medicaid. Nearly 60 percent of those whose applications for Medicaid are denied, are denied because of problems with paperwork or documentation.

Insurance bureaucracy has become so convoluted that it is no longer just the uninitiated patient who doesn't understand. The jargon has become so abstruse that it is like a foreign language, peppered with English words but otherwise unintelligible. The *New England Journal of Medicine* cited this example: "When the Nonavailability Statement is on file in the patient record at the hospital, a rubber stamp indicating 'DD1251 IS ON FILE' may be stamped on the claim form (HCFA 1500/CHAMPUS 501 or FORM 500) since, unlike the UB-82, there is no item number to indicate a code...." If your eyes glazed over, you're hardly alone. But for patients seeking reimbursement or health-care providers seeking payment, such jargon can amount to anguish.

In the current debate on health-care reform, it's worth noting that private insurers launched their politics of reform before the Clintons. Threatened by increasing consumer and business agitation to overhaul the system, they tried to steer reform in a favorable direction. They sensed that private insurance might go the way of all flesh. In 1990, the trade group Health Insurance Association of America worked on over 500 pieces of state legislation. They lobbied Congress for increased Medicaid coverage for children. While better Medicaid access might be highly desirable, it would also lessen one of the starkest criticisms of the current system endorsed by HIAA and do so at taxpayer expense. Another self-serving position taken by HIAA was a shift in its stance forcing employers to buy health insurance. HIAA endorsed the view that employers be made to pick up at least part of the tab. Instead of a downward pressure on health insurance costs if individuals were forced to pick up the tab, this would encourage the impression that health insurance was free. Public pressure to dampen costs would be muted.

It's also worth noting that one of the most burdensome features of our current insurance system has been its effect on the job market. People chose and stayed in jobs they didn't want simply to get health insurance, a phenomenon known as "job-lock." Employers used part-time or contract workers to avoid the burden of health insurance, a practice that increased during economic hard times. Marginal, low-paid workers were far more likely to be left out in the cold than the CEO making millions.

While current reform efforts may reduce the effects on the job market in general, the health insurance changes already under way are starting to skew the health-provider job market in new ways. Through negotiating clout, large employers and managed-care plans reward certain doctors and hospitals by funneling business their way. These may be truly cost-efficient providers, but they may also be the ones who don't balk at "corporate culture." Doctors who quarrel with the terms of the managed-care plans in their area may relocate or go out of business. Just as insurers show little compassion for patients, they are unlikely to be more flexible with physicians. Insurers may force a doctor who feels that he cannot practice good medicine if made to see six patients an hour instead of three, to choose between earning a living or practicing good medicine.

By financing the growth of expensive high-tech medicine but choosing to limit costs by casting millions of Americans into the void of uninsurance, health insurers created enormous instability. They helped underwrite the advances that vastly improved diagnosis and treatment. They also turned these advances into instruments of exclusion, into evidence of uninsurability.

Now, with the help of politicians and public relations, the industry is rising phoenixlike from the ashes of criticism. Under the rubric of managed care, insurers promise cost-efficient, high-quality care to all. History should make us think twice about the transformation.

CHAPTER 4

Losing the Family Doctor

OVER THE PAST DECADES, patients have increasingly bemoaned the loss of the family doctor, the one who would talk to you and make house calls. The world that William Carlos Williams, physician and poet, described in *The Doctor Stories* has just about vanished. It was a world in which patients and doctors shared the human condition. "Even when the patients knew me well, and trusted me a lot," Williams said, "I could sense their fear, their skepticism. And why not? I could sense my own worries, my own doubts." While the general practitioner from Rutherford, New Jersey, was never a typical doctor, he embodied the satisfactions that physicians once sought in their medical careers even if they couldn't express them in writing. The general practitioner whose soul is nourished by the intimacies of his patients became extinct because of the preeminence of technology, the rise of insurance hassles, and the specter of malpractice.

The dwindling satisfactions of primary care and the financial incentives to practice procedure-based medicine have encouraged doctors in the United States to become specialists. Whereas Canada has a 50–50 mix of primary care and specialist physicians, and Britain has a 70–30 mix, here, only 30 percent of doctors are generalists, reflecting the declining appeal of primary care.

Interest in primary care has shrunk dramatically. Whereas more than one third of medical students chose primary care in 1982, less than one fourth did so in 1989. These data fail to show the true decline, however, because a growing percentage of those who choose primary care residencies, such as pediatrics or internal medicine, are choosing to enter subspecialties later on, such as gastroenterology or cardiology. Because of skewed compensation rates that can pay doctors more for doing a half-hour procedure than taking care of patients all day, even those specialists who like general medicine are drawn by the pull of doing procedures.

The most recent data suggest that fewer than a fifth of today's graduates want primary care careers. Internal medicine training programs are drawing fewer graduates of American medical schools, instead filling vacancies with foreign medical graduates—and studies show that these doctors are less likely than their American counterparts to practice primary care after training.

Compensation partly explains why interest in primary care has plummeted. While the net income of cardiovascular surgeons in 1989 averaged nearly $300,000, that of internists was close to $100,000. Without the reimbursement schedules okayed—if not devised—by insurers, this gap of $200,000 a year would never have evolved.

The gap between surgical specialist and primary-care giver might be even greater if doctors received what they billed, which is often more than what they are actually paid. Patients who thank the surgeon for accepting insurance don't generally realize the gross disparity in income, often wondering why the GP won't accept assignment. One study using income projections (based on charges rather than actual payments) estimated that pediatricians would have earned $71,000 whereas thoracic surgeons would have earned $934,000 in 1992. The thoracic surgeons could afford to accept the "discounted" fees that insurance paid.

But it isn't just private insurers who have helped create the great income divide—and with it the overwhelming incentive to perform as many procedures as possible. The federal government has endorsed the system too. If doctors were reimbursed according to the 1992 Medicare fee schedule, the researchers found that pediatricians would have earned $35,000 and thoracic surgeons $241,000.

With fees such as the $9.20 for a brief office visit that Medicare allowed a general internist who had practiced in Boise, Idaho, for twenty-six years, it's little wonder that generalists are calling it quits and advising others not to pursue what they once enjoyed. The $9.20 was the fee allowed by Medicare after its new reimbursement rates went into effect, rates designed to equalize the disparity between surgical and nonsurgical fields. The internist said that about half of his colleagues had also given up their Boise practices. In Georgia, about a fifth of general internists have left practice, according to the American College of Physicians, an organization of internists. A major fault line of compensation has occurred across the divide between surgical specialties and non-surgical primary care—regardless of who pays.

But income isn't the only issue. In fact, it may not even be the major one for many doctors. Careers, like those in the arts, publishing, and politics, are driven by incentives other than money. The bait can be glamour or intellectual stimulation. But in medicine, primary care ranks low both in prestige and money. A generalist becomes defined by the absence of specialization, not the presence of breadth of knowledge.

The generalist also gets more than his fair share of bureaucratic hassles with insurance companies. Instead of being intellectually nourished by the human side of practice, the generalist is increasingly gazing at bureaucratic hassles and corporate managed care. A Louis Harris survey of more than 1,000 doctors found that over two thirds listed the hassle factor as a "very serious" problem, more serious than worries about fees or malpractice. U.S. doctors are said to be the most regulated physicians in the world.

The growth of managed care has worsened the problem, something that many health-care reformers seem not to understand. General physicians are now viewed as "gatekeepers." Unlike the general practitioner of the past whose life was interwoven with that of his community, today's primary care physician finds himself tangled in a web of insurance regulations and heavy-handed corporate rules. The Boise internists blamed their exodus not only on low reimbursement rates but also on problems with Medicare's utilization review. They cited hassles with a local, private oversight firm named HealthCare Compare. The company, under government contract to review Medicare claims, routinely sent letters stating that the care delivered had been unnecessary, according to some internists.

In the world of "managed care," generalists, who often selected their field because they like spending time with patients and talking to them, are meant to cut costs not just by paring down referrals to high-priced specialists but also by seeing an increasing volume of patients, so that more people can join the plan. One New York HMO uses a computer to schedule patients every fifteen minutes, regardless of the illness. Since the HMO also has a policy that anyone who insists on walking in without an appointment must also be seen, doctors say that they may be seeing one patient every ten minutes for five hours at a stretch.

While that is possible if most complaints are minor, it can tax both patient and physician if there is something that needs more time. Although you could find a new breast lump and refer a woman for mammography within ten minutes, most patients and doctors would want the time to discuss the likelihood of cancer and possible treatment options. They would also want time for comforting words, for reassurance. While some HMOs involve doctors in their policy decisions, many do not.

An analysis of medical students' choices backs up the idea that lower pay is not the sole factor deterring them from primary care. But coupling the vast pay differential with low prestige has clearly taken its toll. Even though "good income" was listed as a low priority in the selection of medical specialties, according to a 1989 Association of American Medical Colleges Graduation Questionnaire, more and more students are choosing higher-paid specialties. One might assume that their indifference to income was feigned or that they changed their minds as economic reality dawned. But there is another explanation. Students often see dispirited role models when they see generalists. They may be more aware of lower morale than lower income when it comes to avoiding careers in general medicine.

As prominent internist Robert Petersdorf put it, generalists suffer from the Rodney Dangerfield syndrome: they get no respect. The academic medical community, the media, those who set compensation standards in the insurance industry, the public—all have taken the view that primary care requires less skill than specialty care. Added to this is a markedly lower pay scale and a lion's share of paperwork. The message has been taken to heart by primary-care physicians.

The routing of generalists as the mainstay of doctoring has serious implications for how medicine is practiced. Patients are likely to lose those doctors who were drawn to medicine because they enjoyed being generalists. Our system is likely to suffer financial consequences, not just because specialists charge more, but because they think differently—they tend to order more tests when evaluating similar diseases among similar patients. The same factors that make a generalist interested in talking to you may influence his medical style, independently of where he was trained or whether he works fee-for-service. A study of more than 20,000 patients who were treated by family physicians, general internists, and internists specializing in either cardiology or endocrinology found that specialization was directly correlated with use of resources. Family physicians tended to write fewer prescriptions, hospitalize their patients less, and order fewer tests than general internists, who ordered fewer services than cardiologists or endocrinologists. It's not just pay incentives. Generalists and specialists have different outlooks. Generalists may be more comfortable with a wait-and-see approach, believing—correctly—that many illnesses get better without treatment.

Under health-care reform, it is possible that patients will gain easier and cheaper access to their primary-care doctors, since every plan features ready accessibility to the gatekeeper. But the gatekeeper may not be the family doctor they had in mind. The gatekeeper may only be available nine to five, after which another doctor is on call for the HMO. The gatekeeper may have only a short-term relationship with patients and so be unable to resolve problems over the phone.

But in the new world of managed care, losing the family doctor may also mean losing your advocate in the health-care system. Regardless of whether doctors are salaried or functionally employed by insurance companies (because their income depends on insurers rather than patients), doctors may not have enough financial independence to say no to the new pied pipers of medicine. Under the old system, in which the main tie was between doctor and patient, a doctor would ordinarily have gone to bat for his patients, even fudging a diagnosis to secure payment. Many women have had routine mammograms paid for because doctors listed fibrocystic disease as the indication. But it is more questionable whether doctors will bend the rules if it means losing their jobs or main source of revenue. The fewer alternatives they have, particularly if only a few managed-care networks dominate the region, the more constrained they will be. Reining in the freedom of doctors may be cheered by patients who view them as overpaid and imperious. But patients should wonder about the longer-term implications.

Compared to practice in many other countries, all of which have some form of national health-care system, our country offers its physicians shrinking clinical autonomy. This bodes ill for patients, who hope that physicians will defend their interests if it comes to seeking special care. Those with the highest degree of medical training and with the greatest sense of professional obligation are increasingly under the thumb of administrators, marketers, businessmen, and government bureaucrats. Medical ethics cannot stand up indefinitely to economic and regulatory pressures.

CHAPTER 5

Privacy—Threatened by Computers and Commerce

Nine thousand employees of a large Philadelphia company were asked to sign a release of their medical records. Anyone who has ever filed an insurance claim knows that's a condition of reimbursement. But this was different. It essentially gave the employer (a self-insured company) unlimited access to employees' private lives. The release read:

> To all physicians, surgeons and other medical practitioners, all hospitals, clinics and other health care delivery facilities, all insurance carriers, insurance data service organizations and health maintenance organizations, all pension and welfare fund administrators, my current employer, all of my former employers and all other persons, agencies or entities who may have records or evidence relating to my physical or mental condition: I hereby authorize release and delivery of any information, records or documents (confidential or otherwise) with respect to my health and health history that you, or any of you, now have or hereafter obtain to the administrator of any employee benefit plan sponsored by Strawbridge & Clothier, any provider of health care benefits offered or financed through a benefit plan sponsored by Strawbridge & Clothier, and any insurance company providing coverage through any benefit plan sponsored by Strawbridge & Clothier.

Yet the company did not do this to gain access to employee records but rather to ease the transition from a cumbersome

47

paper-based claims system to a cost-efficient electronic system—a move that is advocated by most health-care reformers.

Initially, many of the employees questioned the release, according to David Strawbridge, the company's vice president of personnel, who said sympathetically that he thought that "their concerns were very legitimate." But this was the release that company lawyers had told management was needed. Twelve employees refused to sign, according to a local newspaper report. They were asked to sign a letter releasing the company of responsibility if medical insurance claims were denied.

Patients have lost their medical privacy, on an alarming scale. Most don't know it, and many seem not to care unless their imagination leads them to the possible end points.

If you talked about the loss of patient privacy twenty years ago, people would have thought about privacy in a physical sense. Doctors notoriously failed to draw curtains around hospital patients during physical exams or lower their voices when talking about sensitive information. But patient advocates helped sensitize medical staff to patients' feelings, and architects have designed hospitals with smaller rooms that more readily protect patients' privacy. That problem isn't entirely solved, but behavior and facilities are certainly better.

Today's new threat to patient privacy is insidious and ubiquitous. It takes you unaware. It comes from the computerization of medical records and from the profit-driven trafficking in confidential personal information. Computerizing medical information may allow providers, insurers, and researchers to use overlapping data at lower cost, but it also centralizes massive amounts of private information. Profit-driven trafficking occurs both licitly and illicitly, by companies whose business is selling data and by individuals taking money for inside information.

"It's clear that personal information has enormous commercial value, and the more personal the greater the value," said Marc Rotenberg, director of Computer Professionals for Social Responsibility and a law professor at Georgetown University. "There are probably a lot of employers who would gladly pay a hundred dollars to have a comprehensive listing of prescription drugs being taken by employee applicants. In some situations the law may even impose an obligation to do that, for example, in the hiring of airline pilots and day-care center workers. But the problem from the privacy viewpoint is that it leaves people almost naked."

The only federal law that protects informational privacy is the Privacy Act of 1974, which protects the privacy of confidential information maintained by the federal government. Some states have laws that guard patient-doctor confidentiality or specific types of medical information like treatment for drug abuse, but there are no federal guarantees. And state laws offer scant protection in an age where medical information is often transmitted across state borders. In addition, most patients sign waivers— although less sweeping than Strawbridge & Clothier's—that give insurance companies access to their entire medical records in return for reimbursement, even records that have nothing to do with the claim being filed.

Mary Culnan, a privacy expert who is an associate business professor at Georgetown University, said that "in the U.S, the big thrust in terms of legislation has been protecting citizens from the government." Protection in the private sector is sporadic at best. Personal data from videotape rentals, cable TV viewing, and credit reports are protected, but information from doctors and pharmacists is not. Culnan attributed the sectored protection to specific lobbying efforts. Federal legislation legally shields you from being called more than once by a telemarketer, but which drugs you take for depression enters the computer highways of America. You can rent pornographic videotapes without worrying about bondage catalogs arriving in the mail, but your employer can learn that you were hospitalized for alcohol detoxification.

Although computer hackers *have* broken into electronically stored patient files, the real problem with confidentiality of computerized records comes not from the hackers, according to a Capitol Hill staffer who wishes to remain anonymous, but from the illegal use of information by insiders who sell the information to anyone wanting to buy it—like private detectives, lawyers, employers, or the media.

A report on the National Crime Information Center, the computerized database maintained by the FBI, supports this staffer's analysis. If the system is not designed so that each person who can access it must have a unique identifier, many people wind up being able to access files anonymously and without accountability—a feature of many computerized medical records today. Some people in the NCIC study gained access to sensitive criminal files using the names of months, "XYZ," or the keyboard space bar as passwords. The report, by the General Accounting Office, found that "the more transactions there are involved in an activity, the greater the chances of noncompliance with policies due to errors, irregularities, and abuse." Privacy experts caution against the use of social security numbers if we get "health security cards." A recent report by the Office of Technology Assessment warned that "the use of the social security number as a unique patient identifier has far-reaching ramifications for individual health-care information privacy that should be carefully considered before it is used for that purpose."

If only because of population growth and new medical technologies, one can assume that computerized medical transactions will soar. In the NCIC database in 1967, the year the system started, there were 2 million transactions. By 1993, there were 1.2 million a day. The NCIC study documented misuse that included persons seeking information on political opponents, neighbors, and friends. In one case a former Arizona law enforcement agent used the network to track down and murder his former girlfriend. In another case, a woman in Pennsylvania did background searches on clients of her drug-dealing boyfriend to make sure he wouldn't be selling to undercover cops.

Medical information is also likely to be misused, according to the OTA study. "Anecdotal evidence in this country, and formal investigative work overseas, indicates that abuse of information, and specifically medical information, is widespread," the report noted. Such misuse can harm someone's marriage, employment, financial status, political career, and their intangible sense of self.

A nationalized, computerized medical system stands to be a privacy nightmare, one that could undermine the entire presumption of confidentiality of patient-physician communication. But electronic highways that transfer medical data are growing in both the for-profit and the nonprofit sectors even before a national policy is developed. The National Electronic Information Network, based in Secaucus, New Jersey, said in mid-1993 that its Healthcare Information Network was up and running in nine states. Users included Aetna, Travelers, Cigna, Pacificare Health Systems, John Hancock, Metropolitan, and Prudential. Information that could be transmitted included insurance eligibility, benefits, authorizations, referrals, and clinical information. CIS Technologies Inc., a publicly traded company in Tulsa, Oklahoma, that acts as a paperless clearinghouse for hospital claims in thirty-two states, reports that it has seen its revenues grow from roughly $100,000 to more than $30 million.

The Wisconsin Health Information Network in Milwaukee ran

a pilot study to coordinate preauthorization reviews, health-care providers, employers, banks, and insurance companies. The sixty-nine Blue Cross and Blue Shield plans nationwide have developed a massive computer link that processes 425 million claims electronically a year. They originally estimated that the system would slice $5 million off their computer bills, but that is currently being evaluated, according to spokeswoman Cheryl Van Tilburg. During the 1992 presidential campaign, both George Bush and Bill Clinton advocated computerization of medical records. The Medical and Health Insurance Information Act of 1992, a bill proposed by Senator Christopher Bond at the urging of President Bush, would have required electronic claims submissions. Its proponents claimed that $24 billion might be saved each year. The plan envisioned patients carrying electronic data cards that would make health records and insurance data immediately available. In order for companies to develop pilot programs for Medicare recipients, the administration proposed making Medicare data available to anyone seeking it under the Freedom of Information Act. Although patient names would be deleted, hospitals and physicians would be identified so that insurers, employers, and managed-care plans could choose whom they wanted to work with.

A voluntary task force that was created in 1991, the Workgroup for Electronic Data Interchange, that involves insurers, government, the American Medical Association, and others, called for national legislation that would mandate a medical electronic highway. It is cochaired by two insurance industry executives, the president of the Blue Cross and Blue Shield Association, and a former president of the Travelers Insurance Company. WEDI, as the task force is known, called for the system to be operational by 1994. Although the group suggested drafting federal legislation to protect privacy, this is a difficult thing to do, as the FBI data show. Some involved with the project even say that data could be proprietary, thus creating potential buyers and sellers from the beginning. WEDI, although aware of privacy issues, has suggested that social security numbers might serve as unique identifiers for both patients and individual providers, despite privacy experts' strenuous objections to using social security numbers.

Breach of privacy could make public figures and private citizens vulnerable. Politicians would presumably not welcome press reports of antidepressant therapy; celebrities would not want knowledge of their marital counseling sessions made public; nor would well-known public health officials want their two-pack-a-day cigarette habits publicized. People whose medical conditions have been disclosed against their wishes include presidential candidate Paul Tsongas, whose cancer recurrence was reported during his campaign, and tennis star Arthur Ashe, whose public disclosure of AIDS was forced by a planned newspaper report. It isn't so farfetched to think that those who violently oppose abortion might gain access to a list of abortion patients. Companies could peer at the medical lives of their workers. As a former employee of a large insurance company put it, "We certainly had access to information we shouldn't have had." Most of us want even our innocuous medical problems kept quiet, if for no other reason than we simply regard our privacy as a matter of personal dignity.

But even if a global privacy law were passed, the Capitol Hill staffer said, the battle for confidentiality of such information may be lost. Protective laws would only set a basis for suing if confidentiality was breached. The sheer volume of data being transmitted daily and the huge numbers of people who would have access to it make legal safeguards moot, he added. Rotenberg is equally pessimistic. He feels that a federal law would rarely be enforced, "because it's very expensive to litigate these cases and because the rewards of litigating the loss of privacy are not sufficient. This has led me to the conclusion that if there is going to be substantial privacy protection, it is going to require an ombudsman, an oversight office."

If the pressures to promote medical efficiency and to lower administrative overhead by computerizing medical data are one threat to privacy, another one of equal concern is the use of personal data for marketing purposes.

Consumers have surrendered much private information voluntarily but unknowingly, particularly to in-house pharmaceutical company programs. Johnson & Johnson, a large health-care corporation, used telephone caller identification to compile a list of women who used Serenity pads for urinary incontinence. The list, based on women who called a toll-free number or who availed themselves of other promotional programs, was sold to other companies on a pilot basis. The story came to light, Culnan said, only after Mary Carnevale, a *Wall Street Journal* reporter, picked up on a notice that "a list of Johnson & Johnson adult health responders, complete with demographic enhancements," was being sold. The 5-million-name list, including 1 million from 1993, was advertised in *DM News*, a direct marketing publication. The brief article noted that "while reluctant to disclose the name of the product, Burnett [the company selling the list] spokespersons said it was most often requested by older women." Culnan said that Serenity pads weren't mentioned, probably because of the product's sensitive nature. One can safely say that most women would not want their urinary incontinence to be the basis of a mailing list.

Congressman Edward Markey, who chairs the House subcommittee on telecommunications and finance, asked the company to explain the policy. Ralph Larsen, chairman of Johnson & Johnson, replied: "The only information provided to the listing company was names and addresses; no confidential medical or other information was disclosed." He stated that "companies buying our list do not know that the list is Serenity responders"— although presumably a shrewd marketer could couple the demographic information with the company name to surmise the product. But Larsen conceded that, in accordance with standard direct marketing practices, no consumer was informed that her name and address would be given to a third party.

Pharmaceutical firms are acquiring lists of patients who use their products, and are adapting techniques that have been successful in the consumer market, in which the company builds a direct relationship with customers. Patients, by returning a card with name and address, supply information without being aware of the company's hidden agenda. Marion Merrell Dow offered allergy patients free information about allergies. It then mailed letters to 5 million allergy sufferers about the benefits of its Seldane-D and a table comparing its product to rival preparations. Marion Merrell Dow also sent a newsletter to 350,000 heart patients taking its heart drug Cardizem. The company was looking at new ways to use the mailing list.

A variety of businesses have been created specifically to collect and sell databases. While these were tailored to the deep pockets of the pharmaceutical industry when profits were in the double digits, there is no reason that they couldn't conform to the needs of new enterprises—like the for-profit HMOs that are growing in the current climate of health-care reform.

The major information gatherers are companies involved in dispensing medications—mail-order or retail pharmacies. Ironically, many of these companies which are meant to lower prescription costs have discovered that they can create by-products like mailing lists or physician profiles, which can be sold to drug companies for marketing purposes—thus raising drug costs.

Market research has become an integral part of dispensing medication. Nearly half of the 1.6 billion prescriptions that are filled each year are estimated to enter the marketing-information circuit, which is fed by roughly half of the nation's 60,000 drugstores. The two largest firms that collect this data are IMS International and Walsh International.

IMS was bought by Dun & Bradstreet in 1988, a company that claims to be the world's largest marketer of business information. According to IMS sources, the company filters information from more than 30,000 retail pharmacies for pharmaceutical clients. Each month, data is collected from more than 100 million prescriptions and 600,000 prescribers—including doctors, nurse practitioners, dentists, and others. Through its "Xponent" product, IMS provides prescribing profiles of individual doctors, including their addresses and behavioral data, such as the effects of medical symposia on their prescribing habits.

It doesn't take a rocket scientist to infer patient data from prescriber information. Knowing that patient X sees doctor Y—who is a heavy prescriber of AZT and lithium—someone might infer that patient X is likely to suffer from a serious illness such as AIDS or manic-depressive disorder. That someone could be an insurer, an employer, or a private detective. And Mr. Jones is unlikely to know anything about this.

Walsh International, a market research firm, buys a database from PCS, a unit of the nation's largest drug wholesaler, the San Francisco–based McKesson Corporation. PCS is a prescription drug management company based in Scottsdale, Arizona. As an indication of the huge scale of operations, in 1993, McKesson was awarded a $100 million contract to supply the Department of Defense with prescription drugs. The drug wholesaler can feed its information into the division that tracks pharmacy benefits.

As of 1993, PCS processed payments for 200 million prescriptions a year. Although patient names were deleted, at one point, PCS included each patient's age, sex, and social security number along with the physician's federal ID number. The company states that patient names are removed and identification numbers are "encrypted" to maintain privacy. Proponents of computerizing such massive amounts of detailed information claim that it helps avoid harmful drug-drug interactions, and that it lowers the cost of pharmaceutical benefit plans by verifying insurance eligibility and copayments. Opponents question the potential for invasion of privacy.

PCS was retained by a group of health insurers to set up an electronic information network, akin to the computer systems that serve airlines and retailers. The network aims to pare down the cost of claims administration. But theoretically, insurance claims data could be fed into a parallel database, which theoretically could also be sold. Of interest, PCS won the insurance contract while bidding against such corporate giants as AT&T, IBM, and American Express. There is so much money to be made that multinational diversified companies are bidding for this business. As the health-care industry consolidates, overlaps between financial services companies and insurers increase, making it potentially easier to cross-reference financial and medical information. Primerica bid for the Travelers Corporation, and the Prudential Corporation owns both Prudential Securities and PruCare, its HMO product.

Financial pressure on certain medical industries, like pharmaceuticals, is creating mergers that will also consolidate health information. In what may be a harbinger of the future, Merck, one of the world's two largest drug companies, bought Medco Containment Services, a drug benefits firm designed to lower drug costs for insurers. With personal profits like the $60 million that Medco's chairman, Martin Wygod, stood to collect from the sale, it is clear that consolidation has tremendous financial momentum for individuals as well as corporations. The personal gain possible in these deals is germane to the issue of privacy because it spells out the enormous profits that can be made on the way to creating large databases. While those involved in the deals may have no malicious intent, nevertheless others who eventually have access to the data might.

Medco sells both its own prescription data and data that it buys from other sources, like the American Association of Retired Persons. Merck, now owning Medco, could try to convert patients to its drugs, but some people might find this sort of activity intrusive. Merck is now in a position to approach Medco clients, which include large companies such as General Electric. If GE were to agree that a Merck drug looks cost-effective, Merck-Medco could approach prescribing doctors and say that GE would like them to consider switching drugs. Merck-Medco could also approach patients, reminding them to refill lapsed prescriptions. But where this chain of information leads, from patients and doctors, to employers and pharmaceutical companies, and possibly to other private interests, nobody knows. While neither Medco nor Merck should be singled out for potentially breaching people's privacy, their union—and similar ones—increase the possibility.

The data compiled by managed pharmacy plans are quite extensive. One doctor was queried about a patient's use of narcotics and received, to jog his memory, a computer printout of the patient's prescriptions. But the printout did more than that. It offered a lode of very personal information: address, social security number, date of birth, the names and birth dates of spouse and children. The prescriptions over the past year were listed for every family member, along with the dates and pharmacies where they were filled. The Drug Enforcement Administration number of each doctor was listed. Everything and everyone in this patient's prescribing universe had been compiled by a private company—without oversight.

At the end of the printout there was a summary that would be useful to the pharmaceutical and managed-care companies: the number of brand-name prescriptions, the number of generics, the number of new prescriptions and refills, and the number of narcotic prescriptions.

While collecting information from pharmacies and drug benefit plans is well established, companies also arose to collect data from physicians' offices. They generally offered to computerize physicians' offices in exchange for aggregate data.

Physician Computer Network, a publicly traded company, offered to install office management software and IBM computers for free. Doctors paid a monthly fee for software support. PCN offered doctors a way of coping with patient accounts, billing, and insurance claims without spending several thousand dollars to computerize their offices. For doctors who had little computer or business training and who were increasingly harried by the administrative demands of practice, the PCN offer might have been appealing. To investors, PCN was described as a way of stemming the rising administrative costs of health care while, at the same time, tapping into the $3.1 billion pharmaceutical advertising budget.

In return for the computer hardware and software, physicians were obligated to view pharmaceutical ads each month, input patients' prescriptions along with their diagnoses, and leave the computers on twenty-four hours a day so that PCN could access the data at any time. Physicians were told that patient confidentiality was assured because the data would only be passed on in aggregate. But patients were never informed, and, in fact the company states explicitly that "patient consent to such access is not required or expected to be obtained."

Interviewed by phone, Jack Mortell, PCN's chief financial officer, said that as of 1993, the company had not used any patient data, although they had the right to access it. He strenuously denied that there was even a potential breach of privacy. But it doesn't take much imagination to see that there is ultimately a potential for violating patient confidentiality. In fact, PCN's filing with the Securities and Exchange Commission in 1991 noted that "were the Company to fail to safeguard patient privacy when clinical data is accessed via the Network, the Company could be liable for damages incurred by patients whose privacy is violated thereby."

As of 1992, PCN had linked IBM (which held a 23 percent stake in the company), Roche Biomedical Laboratories, MetPath Laboratories (owned by Corning), several pharmaceutical firms, Empire Blue Cross and Blue Shield, and Voluntary Hospitals of America. PCN earned its revenue by annual fees from each source: Hospitals paid $10,000 and an additional $295 per enrolled physician; Blue Cross paid $650 per primary-care physician and $2,950 for specialists other than cardiologists; Roche Laboratories paid $990 per physician. Computer networks become more valuable both to their users and to their developers as more people sign up. At the same time, the risk to privacy also increases.

Another threat to patient privacy arises from the insurance industry's efforts to limit risk. Increasingly eager to minimize their liability, they collect ever more detailed pictures of would-be subscribers. Insurers generally ask for more information than someone might want to give them. The Medical Information Bureau in Westwood, Massachusetts, keeps records on file for seven years of people who applied for individual health, life, or disability insurance and whose applications were found to have something that might affect health or longevity (the company was designed to meet the needs of life insurers rather than health insurers). The company's brochure outlines tight security measures to guard its data. But the information is available to member insurance companies in the United States and Canada, and can be used by companies selling more than one product. If someone has a record based on his health insurance application, this can be accessed if he then tries to buy life insurance within that seven-year period, according to the company's president, Neil Day. People have the right to request their file and correct it, much as they would with a credit report. According to the company, 15,000 people per year request a copy of their files—of whom 300 then request corrections. By 1992, MIB had records on 15 million people and was adding nearly 3 million a year.

While some information that enters one's health history is clearly wrong, other information can be of dubious significance. In 1990, the Transamerica Occidental Life Insurance Company began surreptitiously screening applicants for cancer with an experimental blood test known as the "tumor-associated anti-gen." After questions from the California Insurance Department, the company started to give applicants a brochure that specified its screening tests. Although standard tumor markers are used if the TAA test is positive, according to the company's medical director, Dr. John Elder, he conceded that the reliability of the investigational test is disputed by cancer experts. Of interest, Transamerica owns a 30 percent stake in Osborn Laboratories, according to Dr. Elder. And Osborn retains exclusive rights to market the tumor-associated antigen test to insurers. Two other insurers, Allstate and State Farm, also have financial stakes in Osborn. A company's hidden financial agenda, such as an economic interest in a laboratory test, can give it added incentive to search out information.

Doctors may have an ethical obligation to protect their patients' privacy, but that isn't true of businesses buying their practices. Baxter International, our country's largest medical and hospital supply company, under its Caremark division, bought stakes in medical group practices, taking over the administrative tasks and letting doctors concentrate on doctoring. Baxter, a $9-billion-a-year company, would own the computer systems and the accounts receivable of the practices it bought. Under a subsidiary, Baxter already owned a mail-order prescription business, women's health centers, and home-care services. Baxter's move is not an isolated phenomenon. In 1988, PhyCor, another firm, started buying equity in group practices. These companies have resources and motives to churn medical data. Unlike physicians, they have neither legal nor ethical obligation to safeguard confidentiality. On a small scale, one South Carolina doctor was unable to sell his practice, so he sold the real estate. The man who bought it, whose business was car salvaging, tried to sell the records that remained in the office back to the patients for $25 each—a perfectly legal maneuver.

Medical progress also carries an inherent threat to confidentiality. Genzyme Corporation, a biotechnology firm, bought several genetic testing labs including Genetic Design Inc., which specializes in paternity and forensic testing, Vivigen, which specializes in prenatal and cancer testing services, and Integrated Genetics. Although genetic testing may be very useful for individuals, the information can easily be used to deny life or health insurance—perhaps even employment. Given that genetic testing requires very sophisticated labs, it is likely that such information will remain more concentrated—and therefore accessible—than routine laboratory information.

The link between employment and health benefits can be another threat. The Americans with Disabilities Act may have offered protection to some people, but most Americans remain unprotected. Confidentiality is often dependent on the discretion of the benefits manager. That insurance claim an employee files comes back to the office in some form—remember, they're paying. In the case of the self-insured company, they're not just footing the bill for the insurance. As insurer and employer rolled into one, they also pay the medical claims. Although some companies may hire an outside firm to administer benefits, some process claims in-house. Even if the claim forms don't carry a descriptive diagnosis but only have the standard ICD number code, it's easy to decode. Just open a ICD reference book. The company may want to know the diagnosis because they would like to unload an expensive employee, or somebody working in the benefits office may just be curious.

If there's a doctor on the premises, confidentiality is also tied to the doctor's sense of loyalty—does patient or employer come first? Who has keys to the medical charts? In my experience as a physician who has worked in several employee health clinics, I would say that confidentiality is generally guarded. But I can remember at least one occasion when I was asked for an employee's HIV status. The company official who asked was not particularly surprised when I refused and said that I preserved the confidentiality of all medical information. Another company might have handled the situation differently.

It has become a brave new world for patient privacy. Even though the impetus for making available patient data is sometimes good—like promoting research and cutting the administrative costs of health care—we should not dismiss the risks. Patient privacy takes on an entirely new dimension in an era in which corporations are trafficking in potentially sensitive data and in which vast amounts of personal information are being computerized. Aggregate data are only the sum of the parts.

PART TWO

PHYSICAL EXAMINATION

IF THE PURPOSE of the chief complaint is to lead the way to a diagnosis, the point of the physical exam is to confirm (or contradict) the first impression. A doctor looks for the objective signs behind the subjective perceptions. As a generalist, he moves head to toe, examining the parts that make up the whole.

Just as a physician looks at the body's different systems, such as the cardiovascular or neurological system, an investigation of what's wrong in American health care must look at the different players that make up our system. Just as the body's distinct organ systems are ultimately linked, so is each player in health care. HMOs, home infusion companies, kidney dialysis firms—to name only a few—ultimately intersect.

While some diseases are localized, others have more far-reaching consequences. Sometimes it's a question of the severity of the illness. For instance, a minor heart attack might have no consequences but the limited destruction of heart muscle. But a massive heart attack could have a ripple effect, like a rock that disturbs a pond's glassy surface. The lungs become filled with fluid because the heart can no longer pump blood adequately—the patient becomes short of breath. The brain could lose circulation—the patient would slip into a coma or suffer a stroke. The kidneys also could suffer from insufficient circulation—kidney failure would ensue.

But some diseases are diffuse by nature, targeting a wide range of organs. Autoimmune diseases, such as lupus, can wreak havoc across a broad range of tissues. The skin can develop a rash, the kidneys can fail, the mind can become deranged, the joints can become arthritic. Diabetes can damage the heart, the kidneys, the small blood vessels throughout the body. These diseases work more like ecological disasters than like isolated events. They destroy different organs, creating a diffuse toxic effect.

When looking at our health-care system, it is helpful to look at the players both as focal and diffuse issues, to gauge what is cause and what is effect, what is isolated and what is linked. It helps us decide which problems are basic and which are derivative. For instance, liver failure could stem from a primary liver disease like viral hepatitis. But liver failure might also be the end result of alcoholism that had caused cirrhosis. If a doctor is worried not just about treating the patient at hand but also about preventing the disease in others, he uses different strategies. The hepatitis B vaccine would prevent one illness and have no effect on the other, even though liver failure is a clinical feature of both diseases.

Whereas the analysis so far has focused on the "chief complaints"—the story of what is wrong—it's now time to move on to look at the players, the entities that actually form the body of our health-care system, and the environment in which they coexist. Like a general doctor's exam, there is always room for looking at something in greater detail. There is always room for laboratory work and for specialty referrals. And a complete exam is usually a broad sweep rather than a highly detailed look at each part. But a generalist's complete exam gives a sense of proportion. Is the patient basically healthy? If not, why not? Where do you go from here?

CHAPTER 6

The Booming New Industries of Health Care

Entrepreneurial zest transformed many health-care services into major new industries during the last decade. What catches the eye immediately is not that these industries control health care, it is that they are new, that they created very lucrative niches. Like a new physical finding on a familiar patient, they are a warning that something has changed. Unlike the old-guard health-care industries, such as pharmaceuticals, these were the nouveau riche players, the brash players of the booming 1980s.

One doctor's tale captures the spirit of these niche enterprises. Although the doctor made a lot of money, he was really a lucky pawn in a good business scheme.

A New York cancer specialist was approached by a colleague in 1988. The colleague, also a cancer specialist, knew a stockbroker in Denver who had suggested a business proposal that was too good to refuse—but not too good to be true. A Georgia-based company called T2 (pronounced T-squared) would help a group of New York doctors create the Greater New York Home Therapeutics, Inc. For 14 percent of gross revenue, T2 would provide the managerial and legal expertise to create this home-infusion company, a business that provides intravenous medications to patients at home. The fifteen New York doctors were cancer and infectious disease specialists—all of whom were to refer their patients to the new company.

For an initial investment of $100 and the liability of a $15,000 loan (arranged by T2), the cancer specialist got his share of the new company's revenue—between $75,000 and $80,000 a year for three years. But the doctors saw a better deal. T2 could buy them

63

out. Their original contract with T2 left the doctors free to discuss a buyout with any company. But, according to the New York oncologist, T2 stipulated that if they talked to anyone else about selling, then T2 would never buy them out.

In 1991, T2 bought out each doctor for $75,000 in cash and $650,000 in T2 stock that couldn't be sold for two years. At one point, before this doctor was able to sell, his stock was worth $3 million. By 1993, when he sold his stock, doctor self-referral (deals in which doctors referred patients to facilities they owned like labs or home-infusion companies) had come under government scrutiny. The cancer specialist sold his stock for $800,000.

This niche player—like several others—eventually hit a brick wall. Such deals came under sharp attack and several states, along with Medicare, began to regulate physician self-referral. But this oncologist felt that neither he nor his colleagues referred patients for unnecessary care, only that he benefited from a business opportunity that could just as easily have gone to someone else. If he hadn't been one of the original investors, someone else would have been. These doctors simply rerouted patients from other home-infusion companies like Caremark. But instead of a big business owning the company, as Baxter once owned Caremark, this time doctors owned it. The problem, as this doctor saw it, wasn't the question of ownership. It was the grossly and arbitrarily inflated price of services. "One didn't see Caremark rejecting $10,000 a month for hyperalimentation," a type of intravenous nutrition, the oncologist said. Nor did one see insurers, including the federal government, balk until late in the game.

These new industries, such as home infusion businesses, were like new physical findings on exam—they held the key to diagnosis. While a patient who complains of fatigue could be depressed or overworked, a new heart murmur would be a tip-off to endocarditis, an infection in the bloodstream that has invaded the heart. The doctor who knows his patient well has an advantage. He knows the murmur wasn't there before, and he can see that Mr. Jones looks different. For anyone who has worked in medicine, these companies are like that new murmur. They are the most obvious sign that something has changed—and that something has gone wrong.

Some of these new industries generate their income from shuffling the standard players of health care: the doctors, patients, hospitals, and pharmaceutical firms. Many sprang up in response to the massive problems that developed as our health-care system grew both costly and unwieldy. Many new players promise to fix a system gone awry. The problem is that these leaders have a different agenda. Saving money is only a selling point. These companies have been the darlings of Wall Street but have perpetuated the problems for Main Street.

Some companies seized the opportunities presented by new technology: home monitors gave a boost to the home infusion industry. Some companies capitalized on specific insurance benefits mandated by states: required coverage for psychiatric treatment and alcoholism gave a boost to psychiatric hospital chains. Some companies sprang up under the banner of cost control: discount mail-order pharmacies and utilization review companies promised to lower costs.

Each found a clever way to make money, invariably by selling products that the deep pockets in health care would pay for. In the private sector, these deep pockets were the insurance and pharmaceutical industries. In the public sector, Medicare and Medicaid spurred the growth. These were the financing engines that drove expansion.

In the end, we developed a host of mini-industries, many of which are known as niche players. These are the ultimate examples of medicine as business, of medicine devoid of commitment to healing. Many of these companies trade on the stock market. The main voice to be heard is that of the investor. These are largely creations of the 1980s, a decade of sharply escalating costs and astute business maneuvers. Patients and doctors found themselves increasingly removed from the decision loop, like stranded pawns on a chess board.

The Home Infusion Industry

One of the hottest industries to crop up was the home infusion industry, a lucrative sector of the umbrella home-care industry. The $3 billion dollar niche is made up of companies providing intravenous chemotherapy, antibiotics, pain control, and nutrition. It was a particularly hot segment of the home health-care industry, an industry that was the fastest-growing sector of the booming health-service industries, expanding roughly 26 percent a year since 1980.

The home infusion industry grew because cost pressures encouraged shortened hospital stays and because there were simultaneous advances in the treatment of chronic diseases such as AIDS and cancer. Without payment by insurers, the home infusion industry would not have blossomed.

The principal companies included Caremark, T2 Medical, Inc., Critical Care America, and Home Nutritional Services. Caremark saw its revenue soar from nearly $350 million in 1987 to more than $1 billion in 1992. A small new player, Curaflex Health Services, entered the field in 1989 and saw its yearly revenue rise from $3.8 million in 1989 to roughly $60 million in 1992. The field was lucrative enough attract buyouts by big players as well. In 1993, W. R. Grace, the world's largest specialty chemicals company, which already owned the nation's largest dialysis chain, bought Home Intensive Care, Inc.—not only for the company's thirteen dialysis clinics but also for its thirty-five home infusion sites.

T2 (named after the two Toms who founded the company, who had been salesmen for Baxter) was started in 1984 and expanded rapidly from its base in Alpharetta, Georgia. Its controversial strategy of developing joint ventures with physicians proved lucrative—for both management and physicians. Typically, the company bought physician-owned facilities from doctors for shares in T2. The doctors would then continue to refer their patients. Within four years of going public in 1988, the company grew from $47 million market capitalization to $1 billion market capitalization. Its annual growth was quoted as ranging from 39 to 105 percent. As of September 1993, the company owned 89 home infusion therapy companies and provided management services to 103 physician-owned infusion therapy companies in 100 cities and 38 states.

But as home infusion companies grew, insurers balked at the high charges they had been reimbursing. Market forces kicked in, but they did so late in the game, well after many who worked in health care had already complained. Insurers finally began to demand discounts. In the early 1990s, Blue Cross/Blue Shield of Massachusetts, citing an average cost of $30,000 per patient for home infusion provided by Critical Care America to its subscribers, put its business out to bid—a move that was challenged in court by several home infusion companies. Soon after, the Blues were paying an average of $14,000 per patient. Other insurers also negotiated discounts. Claiming that home infusion companies were charging way too much for drugs, supplies, and nursing care, several insurers began cutting reimbursements by up to 50 percent. They cited markups such as an infusion company's cost of $3,000 for a month of nutritional services turning into a charge of $15,000 to $18,000. State insurance departments also received complaints about such stratospheric costs as $8,000 for one week of intravenous antibiotic treatment of Lyme disease. In many cases, these inflated costs made patients uninsurable. Patients with Lyme disease found that they couldn't get insurance or could only get it with significant exclusions. The insurance companies that abetted these escalated costs then turned around to protect themselves by excluding the patients they had helped become liabilities.

In response to growing cost pressures, home infusion companies consolidated and diversified. In 1990, T2 acquired Intra-Care, a company that provided infusion therapy in freestanding centers—sort of midway between hospital and home. T2 planned to set up roughly sixty centers by the end of 1992, up from the four centers owned by IntraCare when T2 bought it. At one point, T2 estimated that it was affiliated with 1,000 of the nation's 3,500 clinical oncologists.

T2 also branched out by forming a 50–50 partnership with Tokos Medical Corporation. In 1991, they created Women's Home-care, for home monitoring of premature labor, using uterine monitors supplied by Tokos and the infusion expertise of T2. The obstetrical home-care market was deemed to be in its infancy, with the potential of reaching $3 billion, according to an industry newsletter. T2 also sought diversification by buying a majority interest in two mobile lithotripsy units and planning the purchase of three more. (The units pulverize kidney stones.)

In August 1993, however, T2 started to crash, due to "certain accounting irregularities." Its president and CEO resigned; its treasurer took an administrative leave. Several shareholder lawsuits were filed, noting that insiders had sold stock before the price plummeted. The Department of Health and Human Services was investigating the company for Medicare fraud. The stock had sold for a high of $67 a share in 1992; by September 1993 it was trading at $6.25.

Marketing and Databases

Companies that collect data and market information have formed another niche of extraordinarily high growth. While the deep pockets of the insurance industry underwrote the boom of the home infusion industry, it was the deep pockets of the pharmaceutical industry that underwrote the data and marketing industries. The pharmaceutical industry was estimated to spend 20 percent of its revenue—a total of $12 billion in 1992—on sales and marketing. That's a lot of money to compete for. And it is income that may be threatened by the more consolidated world of managed care.

The companies in this niche collect data either as a primary goal or as a secondary spin-off—like the pharmacies that sell their prescription data. They are freestanding or tied to large businesses. For instance, of the two largest collectors of pharmacy data, Walsh International is an independent British firm, whereas IMS International is owned by Dunn & Bradstreet, a marketing giant that also owns Moody's investor service and Nielsen Media Research. While Walsh International and IMS exist explicitly to collect pharmaceutical data, businesses that computerize pharmacies and doctors' offices compile aggregate data as a sideline. Physician Computer Network, set up to link doctors' offices, insurers, hospitals, and labs, maintains the right to collect aggregate data based on prescribing information from physicians.

An interesting player in the field of converting pharmacy data into marketing is Medical Marketing Group, a company that claims to collect information on the prescribing habits of more than 400,000 individual physicians. The practice of tracing the habits of individual doctors rather than groups, such as cardiologists or dermatologists, is called micromarketing. This targeted marketing is billed as a way to make better use of the sales reps who travel from office to office, trying to persuade doctors to dispense their company's drugs.

Medical Marketing Group was an offshoot of Medco Containment Services, which managed prescription drug benefits for 33 million people and was able to channel information from both mail-order and retail pharmacies into Medical Marketing Group.

Medical Marketing Group sold its data to more than twenty pharmaceutical firms, along with consulting services intended to increase sales—or, in the words of its promotional literature, to "curb defection and reinforce the physician's historical preference for your product." It also provided drug firms with an "opportunity to create [their] own patient database" that "allows [the firm] to track usage among sales representatives, physicians and patients."

Both companies were very profitable. Medical Marketing Group's revenue grew 166 percent in 1992; Medco's revenue grew

35 percent to $1.81 billion for the year ending June 30, 1992.

In an interesting third generation of companies, Medical Marketing Group spawned a subsidiary called Physician *Micro*marketing Incorporated that aimed to take pharmaceutical marketing one step further, to find out not only what a doctor orders but why he prescribes as he does. The company's literature claims that it will answer the question "Which of the less productive customers [physicians] are 'clonable,' (able to provide [drug companies] with more business if marketed to appropriately)?"

Very close ties remained between Medical Marketing Group and Medco Containment Services. Martin Wygod was chairman of Medical Marketing Group and chairman of Medco. Per Lofberg was president and CEO of Medical Marketing Group and executive vice president at Medco. Medical Marketing Group went public in 1991; Medco went public in 1984.

The relationship between Medco and Medical Marketing Group illustrates the ironies and inconsistencies embedded in our entrepreneurial system. Medco promises to cut costs by forcing discounts and promoting generics. Its financial interests coincide with those of insurers and employers. Medco makes a higher profit from selling generic drugs or drugs for which it has negotiated a steep discount from the manufacturer.

But Medco isn't interested in cutting society's medical bill; it wants to generate maximum profits. To this end, it hires the ex-president of Citibank as its CEO and forms other companies. The profitable Medco, able to collect pharmacy data, spawns Medical Marketing Group, which sells this data to pharmaceutical manufacturers. Medco drives down drug costs, but Medical Marketing Group drives them up. Medco erodes pharmaceutical profit margins by selling discounted drugs, thereby encouraging drug companies to put more money into marketing and advertising so that they can compensate with increased market share.

Efforts to curb costs have also made it more important to evaluate treatment. This concern hasn't been lost on Medco. In addition to saving money, Medco promises to review the effectiveness and appropriateness of therapy. But it takes a leap of faith to believe that a company having a financial stake in selling certain drugs because of variable profit margins can evaluate effectiveness impartially.

The final irony of Medco was its 1993 purchase by Merck. One of the world's most profitable pharmaceutical houses was buying one of the most successful cost-cutters. Coincident with this transaction, Medco bought the outstanding shares of Medical Marketing Group, so Merck would own both a managed prescription drug plan and a pharmaceutical marketing firm.

HMOs and the Managed Care Deliverers

The panacea for surging costs has been purported to be "managed care," a term that reassuringly promises rational, deliberate, cost-efficient medical care. Who actually manages this care is left to the vague recesses of the subconscious. The phrase wafts over worried consumers like an advertisement for perfume that subliminally promises romance, not just a fragrant neck. A recent television advertising campaign for the HMO U.S. Healthcare was devoid of any medical content and featured humorous scenes of work and play instead. The subliminal message is: Join an HMO and you will be protected from the ravages of disease, not just the threat of financial ruin from disease. HMOs promise easy access to a hassle-free system staffed by caring, top quality professionals.

Even some news reports suggest that HMOs will be our salvation. *Newsweek* featured a story on the world of an HMO, FHP International Corporation of Fountain Valley, California. The story carried comforting visuals: a patient having cataract surgery, engulfed by high-tech equipment, and a doctor reviewing CAT scans. The message was that patients need not sacrifice quality for cost. Another photo, of a man talking comfortably with his doctor after a stress test, conveyed that caring staff were equally part of the HMO. In the corridor, two nurses carefully explain something to an elderly woman who is leaning on a cane. No one looks rushed or anxious. Underneath, the caption reads: "'If you need an MRI, you'll get an MRI—trust me': Treating HMO patients in Greater Valley, Calif."

Although managed care can mean anything from requiring second opinions to comprehensive care in a clinic, HMOs are emerging as its major purveyors. In 1993, 95 percent of families were said to be enrolled in some type of managed care, 20 percent in HMOs. Health maintenance organizations package insurer and health providers in one unit, whereas old-style indemnity insurers oversee care by using tools such as required second opinions or prehospital authorizations. Under the old-style arrangement, the insurer and care givers were not otherwise linked, keeping patient relationships with one independent of the other.

Threatened by the rapid expansion of HMOs, traditional in-surers created networks of hospitals, doctors, and labs that, in theory, serve the same purpose. They are reincarnating them-selves as HMOs, albeit with a looser image. Large insurers, who already do business on a national basis, have an advantage of scale, particularly when dealing with multistate employers.

There are of two basic types of HMOs: those with walls and those without. Old-style, not-for-profit HMOs such as Kaiser Permanente have salaried physicians who work in centers that belong to the HMO. These staff- or group-model HMOs are the ones with walls. Many of the newer, for-profit HMOs belong to the class without walls, meaning that they are contractual ar-rangements. The HMO doesn't actually hire the staff or run the facilities. It contracts with health-care providers to deliver care and services for a set, discounted price, creating networks of patients, doctors, laboratories, and hospitals. These are often referred to as IPAs (independent practice associations) and PPOs (preferred provider organizations). Both the closed models and open-ended arrangements, however, are increasingly known by the generic HMO acronym. Roughly 42 million Americans were members of this country's 542 HMOs by July 1993, according to Rich Hamet, director of publications for InterStudy, an HMO research group based in Minneapolis.

HMOs have become big business and are enormously profitable for their investors. A five-year contract for handling the health benefits of 800,000 military retirees living in California and Hawaii was valued at $3.5 billion. HMOs bidding for the business were said to have spent millions of dollars pitching their services to the Defense Department.

But it would be a mistake to assume that HMOs only add order and fiscal discipline to the chaos and costs of our current system. Business ethics are not medical ethics. Which predominates will depend on who is running the show. A dispute between a Florida physician and Humana shows how the two can collide. The doctor had signed a contract with Humana stipulating that if he left the HMO to work for a competitor, he would pay Humana $700 for each patient who followed him to the new plan. The doctor left; Humana sued to enforce the contract. The Florida appeals court ruled against the HMO, declaring that "patients are not the property or chattel of an HMO." Physicians who sell their private practices are not allowed to sell their patients, but only their goodwill. As doctors increasingly lose their options of practicing outside these networks, patients may find that doctors have neither the will nor the means to intervene effectively on their behalf. It is one thing to fight for principle if the consequence is a minor dip in income. It is quite another matter if it means losing your entire economic life.

The business face of HMOs is apparent to any potential investor. While HMOs pitch financial frugality to employers and government, they send slick annual reports that describe revenue growth to shareholders. The top-grossing publicly-traded HMO in 1992 was U.S. Healthcare, Inc. with $1.7 billion in sales. The company said that it posted a 63 percent gain in third-quarter earnings in 1993.

Other for-profit HMOs reported similar revenue growth. PacifiCare Health Systems, Inc., which is also traded on the stock market and which became a for-profit company in 1984, boasted a 46 percent increase in net income from 1990 to 1991 based on revenue growth of 27 percent. Foundation Health Corporation, another HMO, more than doubled its net income between 1990 and 1991.

While cost control is managed care's raison d'être, sources outside the managed-care arena are not always sanguine that managed care can deliver on its promise. Some cost savings that HMO proponents claim, may have more to do with risk selection than efficient care. By catering to large employers, HMOs may be drawing a younger, healthier crowd. HMOs can locate in regions that are likely to have lower health-care costs, and they can encourage sick patients to drop out through policies that make treatment inconvenient. Free preventive services touted by HMOs, like routine physicals, vaccinations, and Pap smears, may be more alluring to young, healthy patients than to patients being treated for life-threatening diseases. These sicker patients may choose to avoid HMOs because they fear losing a trusted doctor or being constrained by HMO treatment policies. They show up as expensive care on indemnity plans.

Unlike HMO advocates, researchers writing in academic journals raise questions about the cost-saving potential of HMOs. While maximum benefits if everyone were to enroll in staff-model HMOs were projected to be a 15 percent reduction in costs, savings from universal enrollment in the looser HMOs without walls were estimated to range from none to 4 percent. But it is these looser HMOs—not the ones with walls—that are more popular with Americans.

Government reports are also less optimistic about managed care as a cure for what ails us. A June 1992 Congressional Budget Office memorandum found that "detailed and reliable data on the use and costs of health services provided within managed care organizations are often unavailable." The report concluded that "the growth of managed care does not appear to have affected system-wide costs" and that "at present, based on existing knowledge, it cannot be assumed that further growth of managed care would reduce either the level or the rate of increase of system-wide health-care spending." A report by the General Accounting Office found that managed care "has sometimes achieved one-time savings, but whether it moderates the upward trend of spending is debatable." It's like daylight saving time: You can set the clock ahead an hour, but the day is still twenty-four hours long.

The reasons are varied. Some have to do with new costs involved in generating HMO profits. Early in 1992, U.S. Healthcare requested a 10.7 percent rate increase in New York State. Part of the expenses cited by the company were more than $16 million in royalty fees for 1992 and more than $11 million in royalty fees for 1991, fees that were to be paid to the parent, national company. The New York State insurance department rejected the request because it had not approved the licensing agreement and therefore did not consider the royalty fees legitimate expenses. The licensing fees covered use of the U.S. Healthcare name, logo, and trademark. But some reasons are the same as those that underlie every delivery system of sophisticated health care. Managed care can't control price hikes due to advanced technology, although it can modulate the technology's availability. Where managed care has a cost edge, it is generally by limiting choice and lowering the ratio of providers to patients—two maneuvers that are not well received by patients.

In many cases, a look at premium increases doesn't support the view that HMOs achieve great savings. U.S. Healthcare raised its average premium for non-Medicare members by 17 percent from 1990 to 1991, a rate of increase easily comparable to price hikes in the traditional private insurance market. The same held true for other HMOs. PacifiCare raised premium rates an average of 13 percent for its non-Medicare population between 1990 and 1991.

Foundation Health Corporation, which has different business lines, raised its California HMO premiums by 11 percent from 1990 to 1991, a period during which the cost of health-care services rose only 8.5 percent per member.

As the HMO market tightens, or, as investors say, "matures," these companies are diverting more and more financial energy to marketing. As profit margins slip, the compensatory move is to try boosting market share. U.S. Healthcare spent nearly one fifth of what it paid physicians on advertising campaigns.

HMOs are also diversifying, in the same way that the home infusion industry did as it came under increasing pressure. U.S. Healthcare has several subsidiaries, according to a company spokeswoman. Its Managed Care Coordinators plan develops provider networks for multistate employers. Its U.S. Quality Algorithms, Inc., develops and markets "performance and im-provement measures" to hospitals, managed-care organizations, government organizations, and drug manufacturers and its Workers Comp Advantage program offers a managed-care ap-proach to workers' compensation. PacifiCare began offering new services: LifeLink, "an insurance product for chemical depen-dency and behavioral health," and ChiroCare, a program provid-ing supplemental chiropractic benefits. Foundation Health Corporation, in 1991, bought a California life and disability insurance company.

With workers' compensation claims rising dramatically, the HMO industry will be poised for expansion into this market. Currently eating up $70 billion annually and possibly rising to $120 billion by 1995, workers' comp has been targeted by em-ployers who are looking for ways to rein in costs. Whereas 20 percent of workers' comp costs in the 1970s were due to medical expenses, it's now 50 percent. FHP International Corporation, the HMO based in Fountain Valley, California, already provides workers' comp benefits for roughly sixty employers. Limiting growth in more than half the states, however, are regulations that won't let injured workers be forced to choose physicians from a restricted selection, although this is changing as costs rise.

Even if managed-care companies can deliver lower costs, there is still reason for concern. On at least one occasion, there have been worries about solvency and the adequacy of reserve funds. In May 1992, HMO America Inc.'s stock slid when analysts caught wind of the company's actuarial statement that had been filed with Illinois regulators and that raised questions about the adequacy of the company's loss reserve, the money that it retained to pay future claims.

But a more frequent issue is that many HMOs have agendas that are not publicly known. HMOs often have financial incentives aimed at modifying physician behavior that they don't disclose to patients or potential subscribers. Almost 20 percent of HMOs withhold some part of physician payments that is returned to the doctors if their panel of patients consumes fewer resources than predicted. While the assumption is that this helps guide doctors to more cost-efficient care, the reality is that it is linked to the total price of health care, regardless of efficiency. One New York internist complained when a local HMO withheld payment because of cost overruns due to patients receiving maternity care. He had never even seen some of these patients; they had listed him as their primary-care internist but had gone straight to the obstetrician—as their policy allowed. A pediatrician, when told that the same company had never returned the "withhold" to pediatricians, complained that it was no wonder, given the CEO's multimillion-dollar compensation package.

Many HMOs that use the withhold as an incentive view this system as sharing the financial liability with the doctors, but the practice puts doctors in the position of being insurers. Almost one third of HMOs place a lien on future payments to primary-care physicians for what they deem to be cost overruns. In those HMOs that pay doctors a fixed retainer per patient (known as a capitation plan rather than the traditional fee-for-service), nearly 40 percent of the primary-care doctors must use their capitation fees to pay for outpatient lab tests that they order, according to one study. The authors of the study warn that "as competitive pressures advance," doctors may have trouble refusing to join HMOs, even though they disagree with their medical ground rules. Doctors are not being put in the position of protecting the public good by limiting access to expensive care. They are being asked to safeguard corporate earnings—either at their expense or at their patients'.

Health reformers have claimed that competition will help patients make better choices. But if the history of HMO advertising is a harbinger of the future, would-be subscribers will have a tough time. HMO advertising has drawn fire for reasons other than the cost it adds to health care. A study of several HMOs found that their advertising was designed to stimulate interest, not provide information. The researchers chided HMOs for using techniques such as giveaways and "associative advertising," in which young attractive women are used to entice. It also criticized HMO advertising for suggesting that benefits are unlimited—something that runs contrary to the cost-conscious philosophy of HMOs. The study suggests that while advertising by physicians may be controversial because of professional standards, advertising by HMOs (which also deliver care) has not come under fire because HMOs are regarded as businesses.

But these reservations about the hidden aspects of HMOs are short-term worries. More worrisome is the unstated long-term implication. As they gain market share, HMOs will have had a growing impact on medical care. They will reduce our options, creating the equivalent of giant stores, like Wal-Marts. The potential economies of scale will draw with them increased clout, with less autonomy for doctor and patient alike.

By regulating which physicians can join HMOs, whether they can practice as specialists or generalists, whether they must be board-certified or not, HMOs increasingly determine who practices what and where. A physician's letter to the *New England Journal of Medicine* described how private doctors in Massachusetts could no longer stay in practice unless they were members of several HMOs. Since HMOs were increasingly limiting their rosters to board-certified doctors—a policy that could eliminate roughly one third of all primary care doctors in that state—residents might find their access to doctors severely curtailed. While some doctors might lack board certification because of quality issues, others simply started practice in a different era.

Despite the much-touted goal of resurrecting the family doctor as the core of medical care, HMOs have further reduced the already-waning appeal of primary-care medicine. Rigid scheduling at staff-model HMOs and the increased hassle factor of IPAs have further eroded the satisfaction of primary-care medicine. Their cost-control strategy has largely centered on making the primary-care doctor a gatekeeper. The family doctor or internist becomes the person to sign referral slips. It is not uncommon for an HMO subscriber to arrive in the primary doctor's office explaining that he is there simply to be referred to a specialist.

HMOs, by definition, set policies. If a patient wants a different treatment, there is the HMO's medical director. If there's a medical dispute, it is the medical director's job to settle it. But as an interview with one regional medical director of a large HMO revealed, it had been many years since she had been a clinician. For years she had worked as an administrator. Whether she had remained up to date with changes in treatment would be anybody's guess. The standards used to choose the arbiter of last appeal vary widely from one plan to another. Most patients would prefer that their medical fates be decided by someone they can see, rather by than a medical Wizard of Oz.

Hospitals and Related Facilities

While nonprofit, inner-city hospitals have struggled to cope with the uninsured, the rise of AIDS, the spread of tuberculosis, and violence-related disease, the for-profit hospital sector has been a source of massive profits. Investors created not only large general hospital chains but also boutique facilities—like psychiatric hospitals, rehabilitation centers, and "subacute" hospitals.

Fueled by Medicare's initial payment system that allowed hospitals to bill their costs plus 6 to 8 percent, hospitals drew the attention of entrepreneurs. For executives, these hospital chains have been enormously lucrative. Dr. Thomas Frist, chairman of the Hospital Corporation of America, was reported to be the nation's highest paid executive in 1992. His total compensation was $127 million. Interestingly, many hospital chains were created by lawyers. Humana was started by two lawyers. Columbia Hospital Corporation, which recently became the largest for-profit chain, was started by a lawyer. National Medical Enterprises, a psychiatric hospital chain, was started by three lawyers. While doctors are routinely chastised for their high wages, entrepreneurs—many of whom are lawyers—have claimed the largest winnings in health care.

The profitability of the for-profit hospital sector might lead one to assume that they are simply more efficient than the nonprofit sector, that they are better equipped to trim inefficiencies. But the explanation probably lies elsewhere. The hospital industry, like the home infusion industry, grew because insurers were willing to pay without close scrutiny and because businessmen carefully pursued the sectors with high profit margins. Several studies done around 1980 found that investor-owned chains had higher profits mainly because of higher use and charges for ancillary services, such as X-rays and blood tests. One analysis found that "administrative costs," which included running corporate headquarters, ran 32 percent higher than those of nonprofit hospitals. An Atlanta hospital owned by HCA had charges that were 35 percent higher than the national average in 1992, according to J.D. Kleinke, a principal with HCIA Inc, a Baltimore health-care research firm.

The story of for-profit hospital chains in the 1980s was one of rapid growth that eventually stalled, often because the chains ran into trouble with Medicare, private insurers, or state insurance departments.

Humana, once a seventy-eight-hospital chain based in Louisville, Kentucky, was started in 1961 by David Jones and Wendell Cherry as a nursing home chain called Extendicare. In 1972, it was transformed to a for-profit hospital chain, and was renamed Humana in 1974. In the 1980s, Humana diversified into health insurance and managed-care programs that covered 1.7 million members. In 1992, Humana announced the creation of three new service companies: to recruit and retain physicians; to offer design and construction advice to hospitals; and to provide technology assessment and management of clinical information services.

Humana ran into trouble with Medicare when the inspector general of Health and Human Services, the government agency that oversees Medicare, claimed that it had submitted $21 million in inappropriate charges for the fiscal year ending August 1990. Although Medicare allows health-care providers to be reimbursed for a part of their home-office and administrative costs, HHS balked at some of Humana's claims: $35,000 for Republican fund-raisers, $22,000 related to alterations on a "Texas stadium suite," and a party celebrating the success of lobbying efforts. Humana acknowledged that $7 million had been inadvertently misreported but defended itself against suggestions that the costs were fraudulent. In a full-page ad in major newspapers, Humana said that because of the complexity of billing (11,000 pages of instructions), disputes were likely to occur. However, citing historical precedent, Humana suggested that it would be vindicated. The company said that its positions had been upheld in 94 percent of appeals since 1977.

Ultimately, the taxpayer contributes much of the revenue of the for-profit hospital chains, both directly and indirectly. Taxpayer money goes directly to Humana through public insurance programs. In 1991, Humana received 30 percent of its hospital revenue from Medicare and Medicaid. Taxpayers also pay indirectly when for-profit hospitals siphon off well-insured patients and leave the charity care to publicly financed hospitals.

While some of Humana's practices came under fire as questionable, other companies were investigated for outright fraud. Psychiatric care and treatment for substance abuse had become big business, accounting for 10 percent of employer health-care costs by 1992. Physical rehabilitation centers were also attractive investments. Both businesses came under state investigations. An investigation in Texas disclosed that some companies had even sent marketers dressed as health-care providers to comb patients' charts for business.

The most embattled company was National Medical Enterprises, Inc., based in Santa Monica and once the nation's second-largest for-profit public hospital chain. In 1992, with annual revenues of $4 billion, National Medical Enterprises owned thirty-five acute-care general hospitals, eighty-two psychiatric and substance-abuse hospitals, and thirty-two rehabilitation facilities. Just how golden the investment opportunity once was can be seen from the founding fathers' earnings—at a time when the company was embroiled in lawsuits and allegations of fraud. In 1993, Richard Eamer sold more than $19 million of NME stock and got a $9 million severance package. Leonard Cohen's compensation was nearly $3 million. And John Bedrosian, who was "relieved of his executive duties" at age fifty-eight, was entitled to collect at least his $510,000 annual salary until age sixty-five.

The company's psychiatric hospitals came under sharp attack by both state authorities and insurance companies. In June 1992, the company paid a $9 million fine as part of a civil settlement with the Texas attorney general. At that time, investigations in Florida and New Jersey were pending. Although the company did not admit wrongdoing, it made certain agreements. It was prohibited from paying Texas public school officials for referrals and from rewarding hospital workers for keeping beds filled. Former employees alleged that "bounty hunter fees" as high as $2,000 had been paid to those in a position to refer patients, including probation officers, clergymen, and officers of corporate employee assistance programs. One former employee even said that he made cold calls to nursery schools.

But the psychiatric division's woes continued. In July 1992, eight insurers filed suit against the company for fraud. The suit, filed in federal court in Washington, sought triple damages for fraudulent claims—claims for treatment that was unnecessary or not provided. The insurers did not state how much of the more than $490 million paid to National Medical Enterprises between 1988 and 1991 was considered fraudulent. A 1993 filing with the Securities and Exchange Commission made public that the company's psychiatric hospitals in Missouri had been added to the list of facilities under investigation. And in August of 1993, hundreds of federal agents raided more than twenty NME facilities. At the end of 1993, National Medical Enterprises paid nearly $90 million to a group of thirteen insurance companies, hoping to end all insurance litigation against the hospital company.

National Medical Enterprises wasn't the only psychiatric hospital chain under fire. Charter Medical Corporation also settled claims brought by the Texas attorney general. Charter, which owned seventy-nine psychiatric hospitals, agreed to pay the state $550,000 for investigation costs, withdraw $1.1 million in claims, and provide $1.6 million worth of psychiatric services to Texas residents for free.

Rehabilitation hospitals were another type of specialized hospital that had a meteoric rise in the 1980s and a controversial endplay. Facilities that catered to head injury caused by either accidents or disease grew from fewer than twenty centers in 1980 to more than seven hundred by 1992. The United States was spending an estimated $25 billion a year on treating head injuries. Other rehabilitation hospitals catered to people without neurological illnesses, like automobile accident victims, who needed to regain mobility after serious injuries. An aging population, suffering from illnesses such as strokes and broken hips, also bolstered the rehab industry, whose revenue was estimated to be as much as $14 billion a year and growing 15 percent annually, according to the National Association of Rehabilitation Facilities in Reston, Virginia. The major players—including National Medical Enterprises, Continental Medical Systems, HealthSouth Rehabilitation, NovaCare/Rehab Systems, and AdvantageHealth Corporation—grew steadily throughout the 1980s.

One company that came under severe attack was New Medico Healthcare System, a privately owned chain of facilities that specialized in treating head-injury patients. The company, based in Lynn, Massachusetts, operated thirty-six centers in fifteen states—before congressional hearings and federal probes began. In 1991, the company's revenue was estimated to be about $400 million. Critics of for-profit head-injury centers reported that patients were discharged once their insurance ran out, after monthly bills that ran to $30,000. A published study found that the average length of stay for New Medico patients was nearly nine months and cost $106,000. New Medico's records were seized by the FBI as part of an investigation that also involved the U.S. Department of Health and Human Services and the Defense Criminal Investigation Services, part of the U.S. Department of Defense.

Although the rehab industry came under repeated attack for "a tendency to overmarket and underserve," an investigation by the same Texas panel that looked into fraud at psychiatric hospitals failed to uncover widespread abuse in the rehab industry.

Another type of hospital also started to grow in the late 1980s. Subacute hospitals were general hospitals minus the high tech. This niche aimed to capture hospitalized but stable patients, such as those undergoing chemotherapy or recovering from burns. Companies included American Transitional Hospitals and Vencor Inc. Other companies are diversifying to join the market. Beverly Enterprises, a nursing home firm in Arkansas, planned to convert 2,000 beds to subacute care, roughly 10 percent of the beds in its 880 nursing homes. Integrated Health Services in Maryland, a company that went public in 1991, saw its quarterly earnings rise from $1.1 million to $2.9 million after converting nursing-home wings to mini-hospitals. The price restrictions that fetter traditional hospitals don't apply to the subacute hospital industry. Medicare flat-rate reimbursements, known as the DRG system of reimbursement, don't apply. And, at least initially, private insurers did not apply price limits. Converting nursing homes to subacute hospitals was relatively cheap and the profits were larger, with margins running between 10 and 20 percent rather than 3 to 5 percent. With annual revenues estimated to be about $1 billion, it is a small fraction of the $300 billion hospital market. Touting it as a way to trim medical costs, enthusiasts say the subacute niche could earn $5 to $7 billion by the turn of the century.

Although they are lucrative, such facilities may not be needed. Many acute-care hospitals have "step-down" units to treat patients coming out of intensive care units. The persistent fragmentation of the health-care market and attempts to skim off the most profitable sectors ultimately result in higher costs: There are more people who want a share of the pie. Many facilities that provide necessary but money-losing services are left in the lurch, unable to retain the profitable services that could offset their losses. Once the insurance constrictions apply to the new sector as they do to the mature ones, it is unlikely to remain so profitable. We are developing facilities based on potential profit rather than medical need.

While the 1980s saw rapid expansion, the story of the 1990s is one of consolidation into giant chains. In October 1993, the two largest hospital chains, Hospital Corporation of America and Columbia Healthcare Inc., agreed to merge, forming a 190-hospital chain with revenues expected to exceed $10 billion a year, the largest investor-owned hospital chain in the world. Columbia Healthcare had only been formed one month earlier, by the merger of Columbia Hospital Corporation with Galen Health Care (the hospital chain spun off by Humana when it separated its HMO from its hospital business). Now Columbia Healthcare was buying HCA for $5.7 billion. A few days after the merger, Columbia signed an agreement with Medical Care America, then the largest provider of outpatient surgery and home infusion care. (Medical Care America had been formed a year before by the merger of Medical Care International and Critical Care America.) Horizontal and vertical integration of health-care businesses was gaining momentum.

Inspired by the emphasis on regional health alliances in the Clinton administration's health-care reform proposal, the founder of Columbia Hospital Corporation, and now president and chief executive officer of the newly merged giant, Richard Scott, a forty-year-old lawyer, planned to expand into local markets. With an eye to offering one-stop shopping for managed-care networks in these alliances, the new company expected to acquire local hospitals, outpatient surgery centers, and home health-care networks.

The situation was summed up by Texas financier Richard Rainwater, who helped finance the start-up of Columbia in 1987, invested in 1988 leveraged buy-out of HCA, and now owns a 3 percent stake in the newly merged giant. Once the Clinton health-care alliances start putting out contracts for bids, "if you don't win the bid, you may have no business," he was quoted as saying in the *Wall Street Journal*.

Whereas unlimited insurance money fueled the growth of hospitals in the 1980s, the pressures of reform are fueling consolidation in the 1990s. Both have worked well for savvy investors. What they have done—and will do—for the public is another matter.

Special Services: A Very Targeted Approach

Kidney dialysis, a life-sustaining technology for patients whose kidneys have failed, is big business in the United States. Rising numbers of dialysis patients and an open checkbook from the federal government combine to fuel enormous profits. What the history of dialysis shows is that government policy has subsidized enormously profitable private businesses and that these businesses have used their efficiencies to boost corporate profits rather than lower medical costs.

In 1972, the Social Security Act was amended to cover treatment of end-stage renal disease (ESRD) under Medicare in either hospitals or outpatient dialysis centers. Chronic kidney disease became the only disease to be specifically protected by legislation. After thirty minutes of discussion in the Senate, the program was created without formal consideration by the appropriate committees in the House or Senate. What is now big business was started by a Senate floor amendment.

By 1991, the dialysis program cost the federal government more than $4.3 billion annually and was growing by $140 million a year. (The total cost for the end-stage kidney program was $5.2 billion in 1991, according to HCFA sources.) While Medicare enrollment has grown by 2 percent annually, the population covered by the ESRD program has grown at 10 percent a year. When Congress created the program, about 10,000 people were eligible. It's now projected that roughly 300,000 people will be eligible by the year 2000. Our rate of dialysis is almost four times the combined European rate.

With 70 percent of dialysis centers now owned by for-profit enterprises, this is clearly a lucrative industry. The rapid growth in facilities has taken place outside of hospital walls, in freestanding centers. While only 11 percent of dialysis patients were treated in freestanding centers in 1973, 62 percent were treated in these centers by 1990. Proprietary facilities were increasing nearly three times faster than the nonprofit centers. Even though the reimbursement rates for dialysis treatments have not kept pace with inflation, the rapid growth in the number of eligible patients and effective cost-cutting measures have more than compensated dialysis providers.

It's not surprising that the dialysis industry anticipates a rosy future. Of $4.5 billion spent on the ESRD program in 1989, more than 80 percent went to foot the bills of patients undergoing dialysis. By 1989, almost 42,000 new patients were being added each year to the ESRD program. By 1991, there were 168,000 patients on dialysis, 28 percent of whom were over age seventy. The fastest-growing group of ESRD patients were those over seventy-five years old, a group that had more than a 40 percent mortality in the first year on dialysis. Based solely on the aging of the population, the number of dialysis patients is likely to grow.

Dialysis treatments are becoming increasingly profitable. In its 1992 "Red Book," a massive compendium of reports on how to lower spending in the Department of Health and Human Services, which oversees the ESRD program, the Office of the Inspector General proposed reducing payments for outpatient dialysis. An audit of a major dialysis chain had shown that costs for each dialysis treatment had gone down from $117 per treatment in 1980 to $89 in 1988. Since Medicare was paying $125 per treatment, the company was reaping a 29 percent profit on each treatment—mostly at taxpayer expense.

With such huge sums at stake, it comes as no surprise that there are lobbyists to protect the industry's interests. One HCFA analyst alluded to the "powerful renal lobby" when describing a proposed cost cut that turned into a cost increase. In 1990, nearing the completion of an audit that would have recommended cutting rates by 5 to 10 percent (but prior to publication of the audit), he said that HCFA's audit was called off and Congress suddenly added section 4201 to its Omnibus Budget Reconciliation Act. Instead of cutting rates, the government increased the rate of each treatment by one dollar.

Dialysis as business is well portrayed by the story of National Medical Care, the largest for-profit dialysis chain. Started in 1968 with the help of two kidney specialists, the company enjoyed a huge growth in revenues, from $9 million in 1971 to $190 million in 1979. The company also owned subsidiaries involved in dialysis: Erika, a company that made dialysis supplies and equipment, and Lifechem, a laboratory that could run lab tests used for dialysis patients. National Medical Care hired top academic kidney experts to run its dialysis centers for compensation packages that, including salary and profit sharing, could reach $400,000 a year—a lot of money in 1980. Some dialysis centers refused to let outside kidney specialists practice at their facilities, even though these facilities had a monopoly on the local dialysis market. In 1984, W. R. Grace, a large diversified corporation that derives most of its profits from chemicals, bought National Medical Care.

That deal paid off handsomely for National Medical Care's

founder, Dr. Constantine Hampers, who remained as chairman of the Grace subsidiary after the company's sale. When he sold his final stake to Grace in 1989 for $11 million, it was with the proviso that he receive a performance-based compensation package for 1990 through 1992. Since earnings over the three-year period exceeded their targets by 55 percent, Dr. Hampers received $26.5 million for the three years, in addition to $874,250 in salary and bonus compensation for 1992.

The case of National Medical Care exemplifies how private enterprise can enlist government support to promote its self-interest. By the late 1970s, the company signed up a lobbyist, John Sears, a lawyer who had been Ronald Reagan's campaign manager. Sears was hired to lobby against a bill before Congress that would have encouraged home dialysis, which costs roughly half what institutional dialysis costs. Opponents of home dialysis argued that institutional dialysis allowed older, sicker patients to be treated and that the results were better. Certainly, institutional dialysis was better for National Medical Care. By the time the bill passed, a specific goal (50 percent) for home dialysis had been deleted.

In 1983, National Medical Care argued strenuously against price setting for each treatment. Even though the government did set rates, National Medical Care deemed business profitable enough to expand from roughly 150 dialysis facilities to 350 by 1992, according to HCFA sources. Although the cost of dialysis went down, according to an audit by Health and Human Services' inspector general, rates did not. The efficiency of business and the economies of scale translated into higher corporate profits, not lower taxpayer costs.

Although dialysis was paid for by a fixed fee for each treatment, actual billings often circumvented the fixed "composite" rate. Extras were billed separately under a fee-for-service arrangement, leaving ample room for growth. A 1990 audit by the inspector general stated that "most of the dialysis providers are being overpaid for...nonroutine drugs and blood which are reimbursed by Medicare outside the composite rate.... We found numerous instances where payments for certain nonroutine drugs and blood generated over a 100 percent profit to the facilities." Their average profit margin on Epogen, a new and expensive biotechnology drug used to treat the chronic anemia of kidney failure, was 40 percent. Dialysis revenues, which grew by 18 percent, were the second fastest growing sector of the health service market in 1991, according to a Census Bureau survey. Since the Census Bureau looked only at the service side of dialysis and not its manufacturing side (which makes all the equipment involved), the reported cost underestimated the true costs of dialysis, according to Thomas Zabelsky, the survey's manager.

Despite concerns about the overall cost of the program and the excessive profit margins of dialysis, HCFA had stopped compiling data about payments to dialysis chains "two to three years ago," according to sources inside the agency during a 1992 phone interview, who refused to supply any past data on specific chains, stating that the only data HCFA had ever collected were solely for internal purposes and, as such, were not accurate enough to release. Given that the End Stage Renal Disease program accounted for roughly $5 billion out of nearly $118 billion in Medicare spending in 1991 (or 4 percent of the total Medicare budget), this alleged lack of bookkeeping is quite amazing.

National Medical Care was the largest player, but it did not have a monopoly. REN Corporation–USA, which also owns and operates dialysis centers, saw an expanding market. The company expected to earn $5 million in 1992, up from $2.2 million in 1991. The company plans to buy or build between thirty-six and forty-two new dialysis centers 1996, at which time it expects to control 7 percent of the market for dialysis patients.

While dialysis has flourished under the protection of government-as-insurer, other industries have managed to grow despite the lack of insurance reimbursement. High-tech infertility centers have emerged even though costs are often borne solely by motivated patients. U.S. insurers have tended to dismiss in vitro fertilization as optional, akin to cosmetic surgery, even though China, with its population explosion, and England, with its cash-strapped National Health Service, have boasted the birth of test-tube babies. Infertility care is estimated to be a $2-billion-a-year business in this country, according to an industry newsletter.

IVF Australia, renamed IVF America when it went public in 1992, is a chain of clinics based in Greenwich, Connecticut, which offers a range of high-tech solutions to infertility patients. Started in 1985 by a group that included doctors and venture capitalists, the company has steadily added clinics. According to published studies, their pregnancy rates are adequate but not stellar. Other for-profit centers have also opened. Pacific Fertility Center, outside San Francisco, was started by two infertility specialists who planned to raise funds for twenty clinics in western states.

But even if the procedures used by for-profit infertility centers are as good as those used by nonprofit medical facilities (and many are), problems still remain. For-profits choose locations on the basis of potential income. In describing how IVF America selects new sites, the company's prospectus states that it "analyzes the available census and demographic data to determine the number of households with women 25 to 44 and income in excess of $35,000." For-profits may also have a financial incentive to overuse procedures, a complaint that has been brought by former staff members. In fairness, however, it should be added that overuse occurs in nonprofits too, albeit for different motives—for example, less-experienced doctors in academic centers may want to gain experience, or researchers may need more cases for their studies.

While nonprofit institutions can also turn a profit on expensive procedures, these profits might be used to subsidize uncompensated services somewhere else in the institution, such as basic research or emergency room care for the indigent. Large academic medical centers that perform in vitro fertilization tend to conduct extensive research to improve the success rate—which at best, runs between 25 and 30 percent. The purpose of investor-owned facilities, on the other hand, is to put profits into individuals' pockets. For-profits clearly use the techniques developed by nonprofits: IVF Australia used the technology developed by Monash University in Melbourne, Australia. IVF America's stock prospectus does, however, state that the company is putting money back into research at Monash University.

For-profits also drive up costs for their nonprofit competitors, when they compete. Their promotional material, particularly when they are competing with nearby nonprofits, recruits patients at other institutions' expense. If the nonprofits are to survive, they must resort to advertising—an added expense.

A host of other specialized services are also emerging as investors plumb the vulnerabilities of the current system and look for lucrative openings. Dovetailing with the need of hospitals and communities to save money, businesses are acting as subcontractors. They provide discrete services like transportation, emergency room staffing, and anesthesia.

Independent transportation systems, both emergency and nonemergency, have sprung up. Local cutbacks by communities have accelerated the trend to privatize ambulance services. American Medical Response, a shell company formed in 1992, acquired four ambulance companies in California, Connecticut, and Delaware and had plans to expand into five additional regions. It claimed to be the first ambulance company to consolidate on a national level. The company attributed its revenue growth to a rise in its nonemergency transportation of the elderly and handicapped and to price hikes for emergency hospital trips. The company justified its higher ambulance charges by saying that it had added advanced medical capabilities. Whereas only one third of ambulance companies were private in the early 1980s, nearly one half were a decade later.

Anesthesia services may be provided by specialized companies. Premier Anesthesia, based in Atlanta, provides services in sixteen states. The company attributed its growth, in part, to the increasingly complicated business climate facing hospitals and physicians—although one large shareholder sued the company, alleging that it had inflated its business prospects.

Overseeing the Mess: Utilization Review

Driven by the need to cut costs, insurers—including private insurance companies, the government, and self-insured employers—spawned a new industry. Utilization review, UR for short, aims to cut costs by approving only necessary care. Their services range from requesting second opinions prior to treatment to approving hospitalizations and orchestrating case management of catastrophic illnesses, like massive brain injury. Who could argue with the goal of providing only appropriate care?

But what emerged was yet another booming health-care industry. Whereas in 1984 only 3 percent of insurance plans were covered by UR, in 1992 roughly 80 percent of plans used UR. By 1992, more than 350 freestanding UR firms had sprung up, in addition to UR divisions of insurance companies. An estimated $7 billion was spent on UR, according to a survey published in the newsletter *Medical Utilization Review*.

Despite this, neither the efficacy nor true cost of UR was known. Seventy percent of employers surveyed didn't know whether UR had had any effect on costs, according to a report by Foster Higgins. And because UR reviewers placed vast demands on health-care providers, hospitals and doctors have had to increase their staffs. UR requests aren't ignored—since they determine whether providers and patients get paid.

Despite the industry's rapid growth, policing of the overseers was scant relative to their power. In 1992, twenty states had no regulation of UR firms—all anyone needed to start a UR business was a telephone. Seven additional states had regulations on the books but not yet in force. In 1990, when only four states had UR regulations, the national Utilization Review Accreditation Commission was developed. Two years later, only forty-two firms had been accredited by URAC. Fees for a two-year accreditation ranged from $5,000 to $11,000—yet another expense added to our health-care system.

Many utilization review companies develop their own criteria, while others buy guidelines from other companies. UR firms generally regard their criteria as proprietary in order to prevent doctors, hospitals, and patients from circumventing the restrictions or "gaming the system," in industry argot. Because of the secrecy, it is difficult to know how good the guidelines are or how well they are applied. If decisions are appealed, it then becomes a matter of somebody's judgment. While written guidelines generally inform the decisions of the first-line reviewers, who are often nurses, there are generally no such formal criteria if decisions are referred to the next level—usually to a doctor. How qualified that doctor is to make the judgment is anyone's guess. The question may not be in their area of expertise or they may not seek a truly expert opinion, according to Sandi Isaacson, a nurse who is now a General Accounting Office evaluator.

UR firms make their money by cutting insurers' expenses, appropriately or otherwise. One of the ironic features of UR is that it often reduces insurers' costs by making the system less rather than more efficient. Reviewers without expert medical knowledge cost doctors, hospitals, and patients a lot of time and aggravation—which ultimately translates into money. Looking at 250,000 cases that had been subject to UR, a study by Value Health Sciences Inc. found that 30 percent were denied when reviewed by nurses. However, when referred on to physician-reviewers, 9 percent were ultimately denied. While proponents of the system highlight the 9 percent denial, critics point out what it costs to save those expenses. Someone has to pay the office staff and the reviewing staff, and to maintain the computerized data. Added to that, is the frustration of patients and their health-care providers, which is sometimes overwhelming. And in the end, many decisions are reversed. In this one example, 52,500 cases were first denied only to be subsequently approved.

If health-care providers pass on their higher costs of doing business, their rising costs are cited as further evidence justifying utilization review. We have created a system of the cat chasing its tail.

The impact of poor UR decisions ranges from annoying to fatal. One internist reported problems hospitalizing a ninety-year-old woman who had recurrent gastrointestinal bleeding. Despite standard tests, he had been unable to identify the source of blood loss. Because she was old and frail, and in consultation with gastrointestinal specialists and the patient's family, he decided not to order an angiogram, an invasive test in which X-rays are taken of blood vessels that are outlined by injecting dye through a catheter which has been threaded up through a cut in the groin.

Having lost about one third of her blood, the patient was hospitalized overnight to be transfused. She needed several units of blood, each unit needing to be given slowly over several hours. In between units, she needed a diuretic to prevent fluid overload, since she also suffered from heart failure. But the utilization reviewers said she didn't need to be hospitalized for a transfusion even though treatment would take at least eighteen hours if all went smoothly. They also said that she hadn't been evaluated, even though she had been evaluated during previous hospitalizations. The medical reality is that it's not always possible to find an answer without torturing someone. Given circumstances like age and general health, a doctor weighs the relative merits of leaving a situation undiagnosed. But the final straw came when the reviewers said that she hadn't been treated with iron, which she needed to rebuild her blood supply. She *had* been treated—with Imferon. But the utilization reviewers hadn't recognized the injectable form of iron, nor had they bothered to consult the compendium of drugs that is available on every hospital floor. The doctor was required to make a formal response to the UR firm.

While complaints from hospitals and doctors appear to have had little impact, other forces, such as liability suits, the rise of HMOs, and doubts about the cost-saving potential of UR firms have begun to work against their power.

Legal rulings have been mixed. A California appellate court recently ruled that employers and insurers could be held legally responsible for inappropriate decisions made because of cost containment efforts. But a Houston court reached a different conclusion. It found that a UR company, United Healthcare Inc., was not liable for malpractice even though denial of hospital authorization had led to the death of an infant. A thirty-six-year-old woman, whose previous pregnancy had been complicated, developed high blood pressure and other complications that are known to jeopardize a pregnancy. Although her obstetrician wanted to hospitalize her toward the end of her pregnancy, United Health Care determined that hospitalization wasn't necessary, that ten hours a day of home nursing would suffice. At thirty-two weeks, the fetus went into distress and died. No nurse was present.

Damages were limited because the mother of the dead infant was insured under an employee benefit plan covered by the federal ERISA legislation. ERISA entitles plaintiffs to the cost of the care they are denied but not to punitive damages or compensation for emotional damages. Even the judge in the Houston case criticized the UR firm's lack of accountability. "Bad medical judgments," the judge said, "will end up being cost-free to the plans that rely on [reviewers] to contain medical costs."

The growth of large managed-care systems may minimize the need for a separate UR industry, since they would be likely to develop treatment guidelines and rely on in-house reviewers if the need arose. Based on managed care's premise of delivering optimum care at controlled costs, it incorporates UR by definition. But even in this climate, some firms are banking on success.

Value Health, Inc., based in Avon, Connecticut, offers utilization review services that are targeted at HMOs, as well as other types of insurers. Its 1991 annual report states that "we have been told that we are one of the fastest growing public companies in the country." The company, which claims to "[Bring] Science to the Art of Managed Care," offers niche utilization review services through its subsidiaries. It offers a pharmacy program, as well as a mental health and substance abuse program. It also offers a "National Foot Care Program" that deals exclusively with "foot and ankle care procedures." According to company literature distributed in 1993, this plan covered more than 400,000 people and included Ford and Chrysler among its customers.

The decision to alter how Medicare cases are reviewed may also deflate the UR industry. Medicare's review organizations—private subcontractors known as physician review organizations—are shifting from a focus on individual physicians to an analysis of practice patterns. This more sophisticated approach will require greater expertise. Medicare also plans to match reviewers with the physicians being reviewed, using like specialists and local physicians. In the past, PROs had often used nurses and physicians from unrelated specialties or different communities to review physician decisions. The new approach will require a more highly trained staff.

But regardless of which medical industry one looks at—whether it's UR, home infusion, or dialysis—one sees enormous adaptability in search of revenue growth. The fluidity of these industries means that advances are quickly brought to the marketplace. But their pure financial agenda means that services are priced at whatever the market will bear and may be of questionable medical benefit. The global health-care picture is not their concern.

CHAPTER 7

The Pharmaceutical Industry

ATTACKS ON THE PROFITEERING of the pharmaceutical manufacturers were the opening salvo in the Clintons' efforts to reform health care. With pharmaceutical profits running in the double digits, and many people, like Medicare recipients, having to pay costs out of pocket, drug firms made obvious whipping boys. Despite the criticism, the drug industry has a genuine role to play in health care, and its has not shirked its fundamental responsibility to provide first-class treatments. This is more than can be said of many other players in health care.

Nevertheless many people don't accept the industry's position that its successes justify its excesses. It's like saying a traffic cop should be paid extra if he averts an auto accident, or a schoolteacher should get a bonus for every kid who goes to college. That's what they do for a living.

Drug manufacturers have argued that they should be paid handsomely because their drugs save money by lowering non-medication costs of disease, such as eliminating surgery or helping people return to work quickly. Even when this is true—and it isn't always—it's a fatuous argument. When drugs save money, that savings could be plugged back into the health-care system rather than removed as corporate profits or perks.

Although there is no question that the pharmaceutical industry has greatly improved medical care, drug prices have become a source of contention. As overall medical costs rise, as more people take more medications for more illnesses, as one of the nation's most profitable industries receives extensive tax benefits, the pricing of drugs comes under increasing scrutiny by consumers, insurers, and health-care reformers.

Although the industry defends itself by citing figures showing that pharmaceutical costs as a percentage of total medical costs are shrinking, the statistics bolster the adage that statistics are more interesting for what they conceal than what they reveal. The Pharmaceutical Manufacturers Association, a trade group, argues that "over the past twenty-five years, outpatient drug costs have declined as a percentage of total health-care costs, from 8.9 percent to 4.8 percent." But drug costs aren't shrinking. It's just that total health-care costs are rising even faster. The industry is far better off with a relatively smaller slice of a bigger pie, just as one would do better earning 5 percent interest on $1 million than 10 percent on $5,000.

From the 1980s through the early 1990s, pharmaceutical companies were the darlings of Wall Street because of their steady earnings. Even when the country was mired in a recession, drug companies saw profits soar. In the first six months of 1991, when the annualized inflation rate was 3.3 percent, that of prescription drugs was 11.2 percent. When the average Fortune 500 company had a 4.6 percent profit margin, the drug industry's average profit margin was 15.5 percent. Merck posted an 18 percent increase in net income during the first half of 1992. Profits dropped into the single digits for major companies by 1993, but mainly because European governments were forcing price cuts.

The financial stamina of drug companies often came from new, expensive drugs which were heavily promoted by the industry. In Germany, drug costs have nearly doubled since 1980 even though the number of prescriptions has remained static. Using information from an annually published book that analyzes 1 in 1,000 of the 770 million prescriptions written for members of the sickness funds (Germany's decentralized but nationalized insurance system), the sharp increase was traced to the use of new, costly drugs rather than price hikes for older medications. For instance, prescriptions for a category of heart and high blood pressure medicines known as ACE-inhibitors were found to have increased 41 percent within a year. In the United States, these drugs, rather than much cheaper ones, are now commonly used for initial treatment of hypertension. One study projected that the cost per year of life saved would be $11,000 using an older type of drug but jump to $72,000 with the newer ACE-inhibitors. (It should, however, be stated that ACE-inhibitors often have fewer side effects than the older class of drugs, providing a better quality of life.)

In addition, the costs of specific drugs have also been attacked. Johnson & Johnson's pricing of its drug levamisole, which is used to treat colon cancer, was called "unconscionable" by a leading cancer expert. The drug has been used for decades by farmers to deworm sheep. One Illinois farmwoman noted the discrepancy between the $14.95 tab for treating her sheep and the $1,500 bill for treating her colon cancer, using a drug with the same active ingredient. When levamisole was reformulated for humans, the price increased between one-hundred- and two-hundredfold.

Pfizer's antibiotic Zithromax, a drug that offered a one-dose cure for chlamydia, a common sexually transmitted infection, had a significant edge over the standard one-week treatment, which patients frequently don't bother to complete. But at a retail cost of $33 compared with only a few dollars for older treatments, many clinics could not afford it. Another drug that was cited for its high pricing was Foscavir, made by Astra. Used to treat an eye infection in AIDS patients, it carried a *wholesale* price of $22,000 a year. Not only was the drug very expensive but patients using it were extremely vulnerable. The industry also drew criticism for profiteering off the U.S. market because some drugs were expensive here but not in other countries. American Home Products' Norplant, a new contraceptive, cost $350 here, whereas it cost as little as $23 abroad.

Although blockbuster drugs are generally new ones, demographic changes are turning some older drugs into big winners. As the baby-boom generation hits menopause, the market for estrogen replacement is expected to soar. Premarin, a fifty-year-old drug used to treat menopausal symptoms, has roughly 75 percent of the U.S. market, according to Wyeth-Ayerst officials. Even if market share remains stable, the company estimates that it could grow into a $1 billion product.

As the number of elderly—and the very old in particular—grows, so does the market for drugs aimed at chronic diseases such as Alzheimer's, arthritis, heart failure, and high blood pressure. Many of today's costly drugs are maintenance drugs; they will be used for life. Even if the prices of individual drugs stabilize, the market is growing.

While the pharmaceutical industry has only recently begun to struggle under the watchful eye of health-care reform in the United States, it has already been targeted by foreign countries as a way of eking savings from rising health-care budgets. Drug costs were recently a focus of parliamentary debate in Canada. Under the North American Free Trade Agreement, Canada was required to repeal a law that limited patent protection on drugs to ten years. Canada would have to conform to the seventeen- to twenty-year patent protection in the United States. Experts estimated this would cost Canadians an extra $800 million a year by the end of the decade, at a time when their health system is also under financial pressures. The extended patent protection could cost Canadians more than $3 billion over the next seventeen years, one American economist testified. More than $1 billion of this would go to Merck, manufacturer of Canada's largest-selling drug, Vasotec, which is used to treat high blood pressure and heart failure.

As drug prices have come under attack, manufacturers have tried to derive their profits increasingly by pushing up market share, trying to offset the pressures of cost control. To do so, they have spent more money on advertising, often promoting "me-too" drugs that offer little and sometimes questionable advantages over drugs made by competitors. The importance of marketing in the pharmaceutical industry was underscored when a marketing executive was promoted to become the next head of Merck. He would have succeeded Merck's long-standing chief, a physician and former researcher. However, the new heir apparent left the company abruptly in 1993.

In addition to the high cost we pay for drugs directly, we also contribute to pharmaceutical profits through tax subsidies, through federally funded research, and through government purchase of drugs under programs such as Medicaid (which spent over $5 billion on drugs in 1991) and the Department of Veterans Affairs.

Under a tax provision designed to stimulate employment in Puerto Rico, twenty-two drug makers received tax credits worth $8.5 billion in the 1980s, according to a report by the General Accounting Office. The law exempted from federal tax the income that mainland corporations earn in Puerto Rico. The GAO report drew national attention for underscoring the huge subsidies given to what was then perhaps the country's most profitable industry. For each Puerto Rican pharmaceutical worker, the tax break for a drug company averaged nearly $71,000 in 1987. But savings could be much higher. The report found, for example, that Pfizer saved $156,400 in taxes per employee in Puerto Rico in 1989. Although the pharmaceutical industry got more than 50 percent of the Puerto Rican tax breaks in 1987, it contributed only 18 percent of the jobs. President Clinton, who proposed phasing out the tax break, subsequently endorsed reinstating $2.6 billion of it because he was told that a repeal might push Puerto Ricans to vote for statehood, which would be embarrassingly rejected by the Senate. The interests of the pharmaceutical industry had been successfully aligned with political concerns.

Pharmaceutical companies also benefited from complicated IRS rules that allowed U.S. companies with operations abroad to deduct a higher percentage of domestic research expenses than treasury regulations generally would have permitted.

Legislation that protected orphan drugs—those developed for rare diseases that affect fewer than 200,000 people—has also been criticized for shielding blockbusters. Under the Orphan Drug Act of 1983, Congress devised incentives to spur development of drugs with little commercial appeal by giving special tax subsidies and patent protection. Under the law, orphan drugs get seven-year marketing protection and tax credits for up to 50 percent of development and marketing costs. A 1984 amendment to the act, however, removed an original stipulation—that companies had to prove that developing a drug would not be profitable. Almost a decade later, 60 drugs had been approved for treatment of 74 illnesses—which are among the 5,000 rare diseases that afflict 20 million Americans.

But many people have been outraged by the revenues these drugs have earned, and feel that this violates the spirit of the law. Blockbusters shouldn't need special protection. Epogen, a drug that fights chronic anemia associated with end-stage kidney disease and AIDS, had sales that totaled $893 million within three years of being licensed. Its annual cost is $4,500 per patient. The Office of the Inspector General estimated that Medicare expenditures could reach $265 million within the first year, of which $100 million would have been profit for the manufacturer, Amgen. The huge profits that the company has reaped from this one product have been subsidized by both the tax subsidy of the Orphan Drug Act and by the 2.9 percent Medicare payroll tax paid by all working Americans.

An orphan drug that raised eyebrows because of its cost for each individual treated is Ceredase, a drug produced by the biotechnology firm Genzyme after nearly two decades of investigational work at the National Institutes of Health. The potential market is estimated to be the 3,000 people who suffer from severe Gaucher's disease, a rare and potentially fatal metabolic disorder. But until recent trials suggesting patients could be treated with doses that were lower than those initially used, Ceredase treatment cost as much as $500,000 *a year*. Drug costs like this can quickly exhaust someone's total insurance benefits, which typically carry a $1 million lifetime cap, assuming one could get insurance for a disease that was so expensive to treat. (A spokeswoman for Genzyme says the company estimates that 5 percent of patients are receiving the drug free.) Sales reached $38 million in 1991, the first year in which it was approved. This was $8 million more than it was estimated Genzyme spent to develop the drug. Genzyme's chief executive, Henri Termeer, was quoted in the *New York Times* as defending high profit margins by saying, "It's like wildcatting in Texas. If there was a cap on how much you could make, you wouldn't get people to drill all the dry holes they need to drill in order to come up with the few winners that carry the company."

Orphan drug manufacturers have drawn fire not just because of profits that violate the spirit of the law or the hidden expense of taxpayer support. Some pharmaceutical firms have been attacked for the artificial way in which they achieved orphan drug status. Using a tactic known as "salami slicing," they carved the potential market into slices thin enough to qualify. Biogen got orphan drug status for its drug beta-interferon several times over: in February 1991 for treatment of metastatic kidney cancer, in April 1991 for treatment of malignant melanoma, two weeks later for treating T-cell lymphoma, and then in May 1991 for treating AIDS-related Kaposi's sarcoma. For each new disease, the 200,000-person limit starts anew. The meter may never stop ticking.

Taxol, an anticancer drug developed by Bristol-Myers Squibb with funding from the government, got approval as an orphan drug for use in treating patients with ovarian cancer. But the drug was known to show promise for other cancers, including advanced lung and breast tumors. According to some financial analysts, the drug is expected to reach sales of $350 million by 1995.

Government health plans also underwrite pharmaceutical profits by paying for drug benefits. Both Medicaid and the Department of Veterans Affairs pay for prescription drugs. Medicaid spending on prescription drugs is estimated to have risen 20 percent a year and accounts for 10 percent of the $67 billion that Americans spend on prescription drugs each year. Needless to say, the pharmaceutical industry vigorously opposed efforts to create Medicaid formularies (restricted lists of drugs), even though such formularies are already used in hospitals and HMOs across the country. The industry went so far as to create the Coalition for Equal Access to Medicines, a coalition of poor and minority people to lobby Congress against legislation that would foster Medicaid formularies. The disenfranchised were thought by the industry to be a more sympathetic group than well-heeled pharmaceutical executives or lobbyists.

Other tax-based programs that contributed to drug profits included the Department of Veterans Affairs, which spent $841 million on pharmacy services in fiscal year 1992. Although Medicare, the federal insurance for the elderly and some disabled people, does not pay for outpatient drugs, it has helped finance some blockbuster drugs, such as the antianemia drug Epogen that is used by kidney dialysis patients.

Pharmaceutical pricing is by far the largest issue when the industry is criticized. But a disturbing role that the drug industry has played in American medicine is its function as physician educator. The role was handed over by the medical profession, which had trouble keeping up with the fast-paced changes. What was cutting-edge during a hospital residency could be obsolete a few years into practice. In reality, doctors often receive their ongoing education in pharmacology from drug companies, not from impartial academic sources.

Although pharmaceutical advertising has been attacked as promotional rather than strictly educational, one can hardly blame the industry for that. Food companies advertise the nutritional benefits of their products, even if another item is vastly superior. But the findings are worrisome because doctors don't automatically receive unbiased education from other sources.

Reviewing more than a hundred full-page ads in leading medical journals, experts found that 92 percent of the ads might not comply with FDA regulations and that 62 percent needed major revisions. Although the study, which appeared in the *Annals of Internal Medicine,* didn't identify the manufacturers, the watchdog group Public Citizen did. It found that most major drug makers made the list. But whether bringing the ads into compliance would have remedied the more basic problem is another matter. It is unlikely that a company would pay to advertise a new, expensive antibiotic and then include the situations in which a cheap generic could be substituted.

The *Annals* study had another troubling aspect. It underscored how much academic medicine has come to rely on pharmaceutical money. Initially, the authors of this study had intended to eliminate as reviewers anyone who had received more than $300 from the drug industry within the previous two years. However, the authors were unable to find enough experts who met this criterion. In the end, over half the reviewers had received more than $5,000 within the previous two years as consulting fees, honoraria, or research funds.

But it's not just doctors who enjoy pharmaceutical money. Medical journals rely on drug company advertising dollars. In 1991, pharmaceutical firms spent roughly $352 million on publication advertising. A study of symposia reports, which are special issues of journals devoted to single topics, found that the drug industry spent $86 million on these in 1988, compared with only $6 million (adjusted for 1988 dollars) in 1975. These special issues are often misleading because they look like regular peer-reviewed issues, but they are not. Journals charged drug firms as much as $100,000 for printing a symposium and charged an average of $15 per reprint—with the numbers of reprints ranging from 100 to 200,000 copies. Continuing medical education activities, designed to keep doctors up-to-date, and often required by professional societies and licensing bodies, also rely on drug industry money, which amounted to $500 million a year.

A mini-industry of trade journals was created to feed on the deep well of pharmaceutical advertising dollars. Whereas the *Annals* study looked at respected peer-reviewed journals, there are an ever-increasing number of "throwaways," controlled-circulation publications that are distributed free to doctors and that are published without academic oversight. Some of these are single-sponsored, meaning that the journal exists solely to promote one company or one product. Others advertise a range of drugs targeted at particular medical audiences, like gynecologists or pediatricians.

The number of periodical takeovers and start-ups shows that publishers had great faith in how much money drug companies were willing and able to spend on advertising. The 1989 purchase of *Medical Tribune* by the large German publisher Axel Springer showed how profitable the American pharmaceutical advertising market was thought to be. *MD* magazine, tailored to lifestyle and travel concerns, was also bought in the late 1980s by the publishers of another trade magazine, *Hospital Practice*. New publications included *Physician's Money Digest* and *Stitches*, a magazine that calls itself "The Journal of Medical Humor." At a time when the recession had pushed down ad revenues for general-interest magazines, pharmaceutical dollars were pouring into medical advertising. Total circulation for medical and surgical journals topped 14 million. Ten million of that total was for nonpaid journals that existed solely to capture pharmaceutical advertising dollars.

A proposed venture by Whittle Communications, using electronic rather than print media, was also designed to gain a piece of the action. In a joint venture with Philips Electronics, Whittle planned a $100 million pilot in which physicians could order samples and request information through interactive videos in their offices. The venture was pegged to a news service beamed into doctors' offices.

An interesting footnote to drug advertising comes from campaigns pitched directly to consumers, which were aimed at the demand rather than supply side. Many drugs promoted directly to the public received very mixed reviews from the medical community, suggesting that doctors sometimes do put the brakes on costly new products if they're not impressed by the results. Recent examples of such direct-to-the-patient campaigns include Habitrol, "The [nicotine] Patch"; Rogaine, a drug for growing hair on balding heads; and Proscar, a drug that shrinks enlarged prostates. Critics point out that ads for nicotine patches downplayed the vital role of concomitant behavioral therapy, and that information about long-term effectiveness is lacking. Critics point out that Rogaine often does not promote enough hair growth to justify its expense. And Proscar was criticized because less than one third of the men in clinical trials reported significant relief of symptoms.

But the industry doesn't like to walk away from what are expected to be high-ticket items. Nicotine patches had been optimistically forecast to be a $1-billion market by 1993. Proscar was forecast to reach annual revenues between $1 billion and $2 billion. Following a critical *New England Journal of Medicine* editorial that questioned Proscar's merits, Merck (its manufacturer) took out full-page ads in the *New York Times* and the *Wall Street Journal* that advised potential patients to discuss treatment options with their doctors, including "recent advances." The picture of a prosperous-looking elderly man holding an infant, perhaps his grandson, carried a subliminal message that one could remain vigorous and in control with treatment. Growing old looked prosperous and leisurely—perhaps because of recent advances in the treatment of prostate enlargement.

Drug companies have also launched subtle marketing campaigns that use generalized treatment issues to camouflage a specific product. Schering-Plough sponsored a national screening program for prostate cancer. Some experts attacked the mass screening program as a publicity stunt. Not only would massive screening be expensive, critics warned, but it is unknown whether screening for prostate cancer saves lives and whether it leads to a lot of unnecessary treatment. The company was promoting a policy that had not been embraced by medical experts. Schering, which makes Estrinyl, a hormone treatment for advanced prostate cancer, countered criticism that its efforts were self-serving by saying that early detection would reduce sales of its drug, which is only used to treat advanced prostate cancers.

Other types of advertising programs that have been attacked include compliance programs, which remind patients to take their medications as prescribed. These programs allow the company to build a direct relationship with patients, thereby creating a mailing list. G.D. Searle launched a compliance program involving its antihypertensive drug Calan SR, ICI Pharma launched one involving its antihypertensive Tenormin, and Stuart Pharmaceuticals ran one involving the antihypertensive Zestril. Critics questioned the efficacy of such programs, and pointed out that they were designed to protect the use of patented medications against inroads being made by lower-cost generics.

But despite the criticism of the pharmaceutical industry—usually for profits seen as profiteering—nobody can deny that drug companies have brought major advances to medicine. Pharmaceutical manufacturers have had ethical lapses—and patients have been hurt by these—but it is also true that the industry generally maintains rigorous scientific standards. Certainly, it's true that drug companies have a vital role to play in any health-care system—something that can't be said for many of the gimmicky new health-care businesses.

CHAPTER 8

The Medical Profession

Much of the medical profession's problems were, at least until recently, self-created. The following story is a case in point.

An internist had taken care of a patient for eight years. The patient happened to be a longtime friend who was dying of widespread cancer. Hospitalized for a fractured femur that had been eaten away by tumor, the patient was in persistent pain prior to the surgery that would straighten his leg. At the request of hospital staff who were uncomfortable with the patient's need for very high-dose narcotics, the internist ordered a consultation by a pain specialist. The specialist, an anesthesiologist by training, used a relatively new therapy, a little pump that the patient could use to self-administer intravenous narcotics. It's called patient-controlled analgesia, or PCA, and is widely used to control pain from chronic diseases or, on a short-term basis, in the postoperative period.

According to the patient's wife, the pain specialist saw the patient once in the hospital, as did the physician assistant who worked with him. Several hours after the pump was hooked up, the patient demanded that the pump be removed. He didn't like being attached to a machine and having a needle under his skin. That was the end of treatment, except for a phone call from the pain specialist warning that the patient would suffer intractable pain. His wife said that shortly after they arrived home, so did the pain specialist's bill for $4,000. That bill may have possibly exceeded the internist's entire charges over the course of his eight-year illness. Finding both the care and the charges outrageous, his wife said that she phoned the pain specialist's office and told them that she wasn't paying. She also called her insurance company to tell them that she did not approve of payment by them either. But

103

in the end, the insurance company—a national carrier—paid $1,000 to the doctor.

When the internist, also outraged at the charges, complained to an oncologist who was more familiar with the field of pain management, the cancer specialist said that he had heard a similar story involving another colleague's patient and the same pain specialist. That patient was being treated at home for unrelenting nerve pain. Several months into her treatment, a bill was sent to her by mistake. Usually the anesthesiologist sent it directly to her insurance company. She too was outraged. The total was $13,000 for one month of pain management.

Nothing rational could justify these charges. The little PCA pump is generally inexpensive. Some manufacturers even donate the pumps, because they make more money selling the disposable tubing through which the medicine flows. The medication was also inexpensive. Morphine is hardly a high-priced drug. Although home care involves some physician's or physician assistant's time, it certainly isn't extensive. The anesthesiologist had discovered a cash cow—and one that insurers were willing to pay for even when patients complained.

For a variety of interwoven reasons, doctors as a professional group (although usually not as individuals) have lost their ethical identity. They have lost sight—and then control—of the big picture. When thinking about doctors, the public is likely to think of someone like the pain doctor, rather than the hard-toiling GP. The crisis of access to care, triggered by the cost of care, has eroded the heart of medicine. Polls suggest a dramatic fall from grace. Whereas in 1960 nearly three quarters of Americans had the highest respect for the profession, by 1989 the number had plummeted to less than a third.

Doctors are no longer seen as a refuge for the weary and sick. Instead their image evokes angst for patients and society at large. Rather than picturing the healing hand, people see the helplessness of illness linked to financial demise. Not only are you sick, you are about to go bankrupt. Doctors have become the messengers not only of disease but of financial pain, if not ruin.

As rising costs force more Americans into the void of the uninsured and underinsured, physicians are seen abandoning whole segments of society, not simply sporadic individuals. Even those with good insurance feel that one day they too might be bankrupted by medical costs. While doctors didn't create the scenario single-handedly, they have done little to stop it. Until recently, the 300,000-member American Medical Association steadfastly opposed a national health plan and lobbied against Medicare. It maintained that nationalized medical care meant inferior care. Until recently, the AMA did not have a high profile in efforts to remedy the situation, and even now, in opposing limits on medical expenditures, has turned away from the reality that health care is eating up too much of the national budget.

In the past many doctors bemoaned the lack of reasonable access but buried their heads in the sand. They hid behind mantras such as "We have the best health-care system in the world." They viewed their job as tending to the patient at hand, not the system. But other doctors exploited the situation. They charged what the market would bear. If you wanted the best facelift, knee surgery, or bypass, they felt that you should be prepared to pay a lot. As with the pain specialist, some created insurance-subsidized scams.

But this didn't mean that doctors were happy with the system, just that they did little to change it. According to a 1991 Louis Harris survey, more than two thirds of U.S. physicians now think that our system needs fundamental changes. Compared to doctors in Canada and Germany, U.S. doctors are far less satisfied with their current system. Although Canadian physicians are often reported to eye the United States longingly, at least one report found that 64 percent think Canada's government-run system offers a better working climate than ours, and 87 percent think that Canadians get better care than U.S. patients.

The great premium placed on specialization and surgical expertise, a practice that could not have evolved if it hadn't been bankrolled by insurers—including the federal government—has caused a severe schism in medicine. The appeal of primary care has plummeted. Family practice has reported one of the steepest declines in interest among freshmen medical students. Interest dropped from 37 percent in 1978 to 16 percent in 1987. Between 1982 and 1989, there was a 37.5 percent decline in U.S. medical school graduates entering primary care, with only slightly more than one out of five students choosing to train as family practitioners, general internists, or general pediatricians. In other countries, generalists make up a much higher percentage of doctors—in Canada, GPs make up 50 percent; in Britain, it's 70 percent. The lack of student influx is compounded by older generalists seeking to retire early. The doctor who wants to practice until his death is a vanishing species.

Money is a key issue, but the great income divide is both problem and symbol. The amount of money you are paid has to do with the type of medicine you practice rather than how hard you work or your level of experience. Surgeons and specialists who do procedures, and generally work fewer hours, earn at least double if not triple the incomes of their generalist colleagues. A once-minor income differential between surgeons and nonsurgical doctors has grown into a gaping chasm.

According to one 1991 survey, cardiothoracic surgeons are at the top of the compensation scale, earning nearly $290,000 a year (some surveys put this closer to $400,000). Orthopedic surgeons and neurosurgeons are next in line, earning roughly $230,000 and $224,000 respectively. Another survey found that radiologists, anesthesiologists, and obstetricians/gynecologists earned more than $200,000 annually. Specialization has become the route to money and respect. It shouldn't surprise anyone that we have spawned a generation of specialists.

Primary-care physicians are at the bottom of the income scale, regardless of which survey is used. Their incomes range roughly from $95,000 to $105,000. These income ranges hold true for private practice as well as HMOs. Surgical specialtists are paid more than twice as much as medical generalists regardless of whether care is "managed" or not. One study found that if doctors were to depend solely on the 1992 Medicare fee schedules, the gulf would be even greater. A chest surgeon would earn roughly $240,000, and a generalist about $40,000. If it were up to the current Medicare schedule, primary-care physicians might disappear entirely.

Medicare tried to redress the disparity of fees (and control costs) by using a new way of calculating fees. Devised by Harvard University academics, the "resource-based relative-value scale," better known as RBRVS, uses a complex mathematical model that factors in amount of work, practice expenses, and malpractice expenses. Its formula purports to create fairer payments. Many primary-care physicians were dubious that RBRVS would significantly narrow the gap. Their skepticism has been justified.

One year after implementation of RBRVS, Health and Human Services suggested a bigger fee hike for surgeons than non-surgeons because of a feature in the new Medicare fee schedule that pegged increases to the volume of services performed. Since surgeons had come in below target, surgical fees would rise by 2.6 percent in 1993 compared with a 0.3 rise for nonsurgical services.

For 1994, the recommendations were that surgical fees rise by 10.2 percent and that primary care fees rise by 6.6 percent. A shift in services toward primary care would mean that primary-care doctors would see their price per service drop. These doctors would have to run faster to stay in place.

A Louis Harris poll conducted six months after the new fee schedule went into effect found that those doctors who spent a greater percentage of their time with Medicare patients were more likely to have seen reimbursements for visits and consultations drop—especially for the routine office visit that is the staple of primary-care medicine. Invasive procedures continued to be compensated at a rate that was two to five times higher than "evaluation and management" fees. Ironically, Louis Harris pollsters paid surgeons and specialists $75 and primary-care doctors $50 to answer the survey evaluating the new payment scheme. The survey had been ordered by the Physician Payment Review Commission, which was created in 1986 to advise Congress on how to control Medicare costs and improve payment to doctors. David Colby, principal policy analyst for PPRC, said that the fee differential was the decision of Harris pollsters, although PPRC considered it justified because "that's the reality of the situation."

Doctors had questioned the fairness of RBRVS from the outset, because realistic numbers were often missing. Physician overhead costs for 1990 were set by using some 1980 statistics because those were the latest available from the Census Bureau. Suburban rent figures were used when urban costs weren't available. New Jersey data were used to calculate New York City expenses. A year after RBRVS went into effect, pathologists, a group that already ranked among medicine's highest-paid physicians, received the largest increase in Medicare payments, according to the 1993 annual report by the Physician Payment Review Commission.

Even for those doing extremely well financially, the uncertainty—and often capriciousness—of reimbursement policies has caused a hoarding mentality. In fact, the Louis Harris poll found that those with the highest incomes—surgeons and other proceduralists—were the most concerned about the new fee schedules (even though they were the most satisfied with practice). While many doctors may have been greedy, others reacted like people threatened with food rationing slated to start next week—they stockpiled. They realized that they would be unable to pass on their costs of doing business, as politicians promised more for less and private insurers followed Medicare's lead.

The great income divide is compounded by the denigration of generalist skills. Not surprisingly, prestige and income are intertwined. HMOs, which have been in the forefront of promoting generalists as gatekeepers, have done much to reinforce a derided image of the generalist. It is not unusual for HMO patients, who cannot see specialists without authorization from their primary-care physicians, to arrive at the internist's office requesting a barrage of specialty referrals for which they need referral slips. Both the HMO and the HMO patients perceive the internist as goalie, blocking access to higher-paid and higher-valued specialists.

When reformers seek to encourage students to choose primary care, they should ask themselves who would want to spend seven years and $100,000 training to be a gatekeeper? Today's medical student looks at his options, not only aware of the great income divide and of the dispirited primary-care role models, but also through the prism of debt. The average medical student now graduates nearly $46,000 in debt. Some owe more than $75,000. One study found that for a growing number of students whose educational debt tops $120,000, they need to start earning an annual income of $266,000 five years after they finish training in order to meet their repayment obligations. Although debt alone doesn't determine career choice, it must make students think about the financial implications of their choice.

But lower incomes and dispirited role models are still not the entire explanation of the flight from primary care. The threat of malpractice suits encourages the use of specialty consults. Some generalists opt for swift referrals, even if confident that they could treat a particular problem. It isn't worth putting themselves at risk in the event of a lawsuit. High-volume practices—the wave of the future—also encourage referrals if gatekeepers don't have time to think about the complicated cases. And some HMOs without walls make it financially impossible for generalists to do the tests that would enable them to keep patients with difficult illnesses. For instance, a plan that doesn't reimburse internists for electrocardiograms might force them to give up patients with heart rhythm disturbances. Because it would no longer be practical to pay for the equipment or staff time, these internists might be forced to shuffle patients straight to the cardiologist. But giving up the difficult cases that are peppered among routine minor illnesses in a general practice destroys the intellectual satisfaction of practice. Generalists find themselves running "well-baby clinics" rather than treating an interesting mix of cases. General-ists are turned into school nurses.

Because primary-care doctors have a higher caseload than specialists or surgeons and because their lower incomes generally don't permit them to hire several staff, they cope with a dis-proportionate share of the hassles generated by both private and public insurers. An indirect sign of their bureaucratic hassles can be gleaned from their overhead costs. A study of group practices found that family practitioners spent the highest percentage of their income as overhead: 54 percent. The time spent coping with hassles—which are usually due to insurance—generates neither job satisfaction nor income. Sometimes they reach Dadaist absur-dity, as in the case of one internist queried by an HMO about the medical necessity of a patient's vacation. The patient had tried to secure a four-month supply of medication because of a projected long-term stay abroad. The HMO's policy limited prescriptions to one-month supplies. In trying to secure the exception, the doctor was asked whether the patient's vacation was medically necessary. The mix of mundane medical problems and exhausting paper-work can make a generalist feel that he is locked in an IRS audit rather than ministering to the sick.

Academic medicine—both at medical schools and teaching hospitals—also promotes specialization. Research rather than clinical skills is the key to academic advancement, a variant of academia's publish-or-perish bias. Obtaining research grants may also be a critical part of one's salary. But the premium on technology-based medicine is prompted by more than a value system. It is encouraged by the economic realities of hospitals. Doctors-in-training are cheap labor. They are needed especially in high-tech areas, like intensive care units. In many programs, if a doctor survives with his desire to become a generalist intact, he will need to learn the appropriate skills *after* residency. Learning to diagnose and treat common problems like a scratched cornea or wax-clogged ear is less likely to be part of training in internal medicine than learning how to thread a catheter into the heart. Doctors don't learn the breadth of skills that would make them truly efficient generalists.

The increasing (and appropriate) shift of medical care to outpatient settings has also had a negative impact on primary-care specialties. Hospitalized patients are sicker than they once were because of efforts to cut hospitalization rates. Not that long ago, diabetic patients were admitted to begin insulin treatment or hypothyroid patients to adjust their thyroid medication. Once the problem was solved, the patient went home. Normal life resumed. Today, most hospitalized medical patients suffer from incurable diseases such as end-stage heart disease or AIDS, or from social problems such as homelessness. Students can contrast the reversible acute illnesses of surgical patients with the chronic debilitated state of hospitalized medical patients. Although dealing with terminal illness is part of medicine, students are likely to feel discouraged if proportionately few people are returned to good health.

The emphasis on specialization and the high technology that goes with it has spawned another trend: entrepreneurship. Doctors saw the big money to be made in certain fields, by creating freestanding "centers." Radiologists bought CAT scanners, MRI machines, and equipment to deliver radiation therapy to cancer patients. Kidney specialists set up dialysis centers. Orthopedists set up sports medicine complexes. Surgeons set up outpatient clinics. Gynecologists created infertility clinics. New technology and entrepreneurship were a marriage made in heaven. But they made strange bedfellows. Some would argue that they never should have become involved. But even those opposed to the partnership are forced to concede that, for better and for worse, the link has made the latest technology available in places that might otherwise have been ignored. Profits and technology diffusion have gone hand in hand.

Doctors as entrepreneurs turned their practices into businesses. They also invested in other medical facilities, like home infusion companies or rehabilitation centers. The latter practice, called physician self-referral, has come under intense public fire. But this is a misnomer. Doctors have always self-referred when they tell patients to come back for follow-up visits. This new "self-referral" is defined as a doctor sending patients to a facility in which "he or she has a financial interest but no professional responsibility," a definition that is more specific than the simple term "self-referral" implies. The AMA watered down their condemnation of the practice, saying that such referrals were okay as long as patients were informed of the doctor's vested interests. This was a disingenuous solution. A cancer patient is unlikely to choose a different radiotherapy facility because his oncologist announces that he has a financial interest in the treatment, even if the information disquiets the patient.

The practice of doctors as investors has drawn sharp criticism, further eroding the profession's moral high ground. Medical practice has always had elements of self-interest, but that self-interest wasn't always economic. Self-interest in academic circles could be prestige or tenure. But entrepreneurship introduced business ethics to medicine. To the extent that "business ethics" is an oxymoron, that is a major problem.

At a conference of neurosurgeons, Robert Blendon, a prominent policy expert who teaches at the Harvard School of Public Health, warned doctors that they would fall even further from grace if they saw themselves as businessmen. "Let me give you a tip," he said. "In polls, businesspeople rate 17 points lower than doctors. The last thing you should want to do is get up in front of an audience and declare yourself to be one of the groups that Americans think are among the sleaziest in the United States."

More than a decade ago, Dr. Arnold Relman, the editor of the *New England Journal of Medicine*, warned of the effects of the "medical-industrial complex," using a turn of phrase that drew an analogy to the defense industry. The analogy was apt. Both industries were vital, and both threatened to serve themselves before serving the nation. Both were heavily subsidized by public funding, as filtered through Congress. Both industries became sources of great personal wealth and job growth. Both became targets of public outrage. Reducing costs also meant large-scale layoffs.

In 1980, Relman cited certain sectors that had benefited from entrepreneurial zeal: proprietary hospitals (revenues of $12 to $13 billion), proprietary nursing homes ($15 billion), home care ($3 billion), proprietary laboratories ($5 to $6 billion). History has shown other sectors, like kidney dialysis, to be major earners as well. Funded by Medicare, the number of people on dialysis jumped from 40 per million to 200 per million. We have the highest dialysis rate in the world. With payment policies that discouraged home dialysis, the rate of home dialysis dropped from 40 percent of patients to 13 percent. The preeminent dialysis company, National Medical Care, was founded by kidney specialists. It grew to include the manufacture of dialysis equipment, not merely the delivery of service, and to provide unrelated services such as obesity treatment. Really big money was now available to doctors—if they went into business.

Relman was an early critic of physician-investors. He suggested that "practicing physicians should derive no financial benefit from the health-care market except their own professional services."

But it was unreasonable to think that doctors would bow out as long as insurers and government endorsed huge profits in the business of medicine. It's one thing to help rein in costs if everyone pitches in. It's quite another simply to help shift profits into someone else's pockets.

The problem that drew government attention was not radiologists earning fortunes from their highly equipped offices, but doctors earning money from facilities where they were solely investors. Attempting to curtail self-referral, state and federal governments moved to ban the practice. Florida and New Jersey were active early on. Congress banned referral of Medicare and Medicaid patients to clinical laboratories owned by referring physicians. But it was a precarious truce in which physicians were distanced from profits that were condoned for business.

While entrepreneurship and self-referral were key issues in the 1980s, physician autonomy is emerging as the chief concern for the profession in the 1990s, as managed care sweeps through the nation. But there are dangers in shifting control of medical care from doctors to insurance companies. It is like flying in a plane in which the pilot is not in control, but merely carries out orders from below. Most of us, while we want our pilots in contact with ground control, would prefer to think that their judgment call is the final word.

Doctors in many instances are not just losing control, they're being forced to assume financial responsibility normally carried by insurance companies for the care, a concept disingenuously termed "risk-sharing." One HMO had written instructions to its primary-care doctors that if doctors did not follow the company's referral policies, "the provider may be financially responsible for the professional services of the referred-to physician." But this HMO was not alone in shifting its potential losses onto the backs of its gatekeeper physicians. In fact, the trend toward paying doctors a fixed monthly fee (known as capitation) rather than fee-for-service carries grave financial risks for individual doctors, or even small groups. As the head of a staff-model HMO commented, an individual doctor with 1,500 to 2,000 patients can't afford to do this. He said that roughly 60,000 patients are needed before capitation becomes a fair way of paying for care. Doctors working under capitation need to spread risk in the same way that insurers do—a solo practitioner can't.

A review of Philadelphia Medicaid patients who had been shifted from fee-for-service plans to HMOs under a plan known as

HealthPASS, found that the financial liability imposed on doctors was too great. Doctors, who were paid a fixed monthly fee that ranged from $5 to $14 per Medicaid patient depending on age and sex, were originally liable to repay as much as $4,000 per patient in specialty referral fees. That meant that for a guaranteed $60 yearly fee for looking after a patient—regardless of how many times the doctor saw him—the doctor assumed a financial liability of $4,000. This was no idle threat, since Medicaid patients are sicker than average because they are poor, and with that comes higher rates of infant mortality, AIDS, heart disease, cancer, and substance abuse. The financial liability was lowered to $1,000— still a deal that many would find unattractive. Not only are generalists being required to "manage" care, they are also being surreptitiously coerced into becoming insurers.

While most doctors chose their careers for reasons other than money, the combined loss of income, prestige, and control is likely to have profound effects. Some areas of medicine will remain out of this downward spiral. Largely it is the business sector—the pharmaceutical, biotech, and HMO industries. Even hospital administrators, regarded as business experts, make very generous salaries. Some administrators of nonprofit hospitals were reported to have annual compensation packages that topped $1 million. The high end will always draw, and there is always likely to be a high end. But those who actually deliver care—especially primary care—are drifting downward. One can only assume that if medical school applications are currently up because other jobs are scarce, the best and the brightest will go elsewhere when they feel there is more of a choice.

CHAPTER 9

The Media

LAPAROSCOPIC GALLBLADDER REMOVAL quickly replaced conventional surgery largely because of popular demand, not because surgeons insisted on it. The media may claim that they are only the purveyors of medical tidings, but they actually help determine medical practice and the country's health-care agenda. Television, radio, newspapers, and magazines bring the latest medical technology into millions of living rooms, whetting the public appetite for the newest and the best.

Televised interviews with elated patients fueled the remaking of gallbladder surgery. Surgeons weren't the ones to make the familiar, conventional gallbladder operation, with its eight-inch scar and six-week recuperation, obsolete. Patients simply refused the older surgery. They shopped around until they found a surgeon who would do the minimally invasive operation. They wanted the surgery that let them leave the hospital in twenty-four hours and return to work within the week. As a result, surgeons had to learn the new technique—and it wasn't so simple. Instead of peering directly into the abdominal cavity, surgeons had to learn how to judge their operative field by watching a TV video monitor. They had to judge depth from a two-dimensional image. Rather than feel internal organs, surgeons now had to manipulate instruments that pierced a closed abdominal cavity. They could no longer feel whether the tissue they were about to cut was hard or soft. If they didn't master the new technique, they simply lost their gallbladder cases.

Media emphasis on newness dovetails with the public's enthusiasm for high-tech, specialty medicine, although few medical consumers link their personal thirst for the latest advance with rising medical bills. A family practitioner interviewed by former CNN reporter Gary Schwitzer said that, following TV reports, he had a surge in requests for MRIs (scans that cost roughly $1,000), and blood tests for prostate-specific antigen and Ca 125 (both markers for cancers that cost about $75 each), as well as a heavily promoted new anti-inflammatory drug.

Like a public relations blitz, the media can make people aware of health issues to which they had given little prior thought. A disease, usually pegged to a celebrity victim or a new technology, can suddenly make headlines. Rock Hudson, Arthur Ashe, and Magic Johnson helped shine momentary spotlights on AIDS. Gilda Radner's death focused the limelight on ovarian cancer. The film *Lorenzo's Oil* focused attention on a rare hereditary disease and on the plight of families searching for their own cures.

Newspapers, television, and magazines can also spark anxiety about health care and disease, affecting policy at both medical and governmental levels. Extensive coverage of a young woman who contracted AIDS through dental work and of medical waste that washed up on beaches are cases in point. Both instances illustrate the hazards of a media blitz. Both cases promoted health policy that was not rooted in science.

Wide media reports of a Florida dentist who ultimately infected six patients with HIV, the virus that causes AIDS, fueled demands that all health-care workers be tested for HIV. Kimberly Bergalis, a victim of the dentist's negligence, was featured repeatedly on TV and in the press as she argued before Congress for mandatory HIV testing of health-care workers. The television cameras captured her transformation from a vibrant, attractive young woman to an ageless, skeletal symbol of the ravages of AIDS.

Her televised plight influenced medical groups, including the Centers for Disease Control and Prevention, to recommend that doctors and dentists doing invasive procedures be tested for HIV infection and that those who were HIV-positive remove themselves from performing invasive procedures. But mandatory screening of health-care workers would have been a costly, impractical policy that would have done nothing to stem the spread of AIDS. Kimberly Bergalis's tragic plight overshadowed a true public health concern, that of infection control. Any dentist's office could pose a threat—regardless of the HIV status of its personnel—if it didn't practice stringent infection control. The key issue is proper cleaning and sterilization of instruments which is boring compared to the media-friendly human interest story.

Widespread coverage of the Bergalis case was a stark reminder that public sentiment, fueled by press coverage, could supersede science as the basis of health policy. In response to the Bergalis case, the CDC drew up a controversial list of invasive procedures that HIV-positive health-care workers were advised not to perform, a list approved by then-Secretary of Health and Human Services Dr. Louis Sullivan. Even though there was no scientific evidence to show that this was an effective way to stem the tide of AIDS, the nation's main infectious disease agency endorsed a policy that had been pushed by media coverage of one case. Although a theoretical risk of transmission from infected worker to patient existed all along, ten years after the epidemic started, only six cases had been reported—and they were all linked to one health-care worker. Some sources have even suggested that the Florida dentist intentionally injected his patients with HIV-infected blood. If such criminal activity did occur, it could have occurred with other deadly toxins. Clearly, something exceptional had happened in the Florida case. The victims of the Florida dentist suffered a tragedy—but the proposed remedy would not have been a solution.

Reporters lost sight of several significant questions that lacked a human face but had far greater medical significance. Given the thousands of health-care workers infected with the virus, why was there a cluster linked to one dentist? Were lapses in infection control to blame rather than the HIV status of the Florida dentist? If this was so, then stringent infection control would make more sense than a witch-hunt for HIV-positive personnel, because patients would be at risk if they were treated anywhere that an infected patient had been treated, regardless of the HIV status of the health-care worker. Given that an estimated 1 in 250 persons in the United States is thought to carry the AIDS virus, this is of major significance. What would have been the rationale for testing health-care workers when the likelihood of transmission was much greater from patient to health-care worker? Yet these abstractions were far less gripping than the sight of an attractive young woman dying before the camera.

Another misguided response followed widespread media reports of medical waste washing up on East Coast beaches in the summer of 1988. This put the heat on Congress, which then passed a law about the disposal of medical waste. But most of what washed up on the beach was not medical waste, just ordinary debris. What was medical came from unregulated users—illegal drug users and those using medical supplies at home. They would never have been subject to the law. In addition, there is not a single documented case of disease caused by contaminated medical products except in an occupational setting. Costly legislation was enacted as a result of media coverage. This waste was an esthetic hazard, not a medical one. In fairness to the press, our legislators could have sought and followed medical advice. They didn't have to follow the media blitz like lemmings to the sea.

Despite the significant role that the media have come to play in our understanding of disease, our view of health care, and the shaping of our health policy, there is little discussion of the biases and values that lurk within media coverage. The media claim to be objective, but every story contains the seeds of bias. Simply declaring a story newsworthy expresses a judgment. And placing a story prominently on a front page or above the fold declares the story more important than if the same story is placed mid-section or at the bottom of a page. A story in the *New York Times* many years ago on the sharp decline in fertility among women over thirty-five was placed prominently on the front page. Many women panicked. The same story, based on a study published in the *New England Journal of Medicine,* would probably not have created a similar stir if the editors had chosen to run it inside the paper.

Leaving a story out or giving it little play is equally a value judgment. While Kimberly Bergalis made front-page news, a subsequent large study refuting the benefits of screening health-care workers for HIV infection did not get the same attention. The study of more than 15,000 patients treated by HIV-positive doctors and dentists—which was done because of the controversy surrounding the Bergalis case—revealed no new cases of worker-to-patient transmission. This finding did not make the front pages. It had no immediate human interest.

Although high physician wages are frequently discussed, a major study in the *New England Journal of Medicine* attracted little notice. The study found that if pediatricians were paid entirely according to the 1992 Medicare fee schedule, they could be expected to earn $35,000 a year—family physicians could be expected to earn $40,000 and general internists $44,000. The study was newsworthy on several accounts. At the time that the study appeared, policy experts were trying to redress the flight out of primary care. While many doctors choose their fields for reasons other than money, knowing that you were headed for a salary of

$35,000 for sixty hours a week, with a debt of $50,000 to $100,000 after seven years of training beyond college, would make even the most dedicated physician think twice about becoming a pediatrician.

But the other reason that this story was newsworthy was that is was written by William Hsiao, the architect of the new Medicare fee schedule known as the resource-based relative-value scale, or RBRVS. Only a few years earlier, Hsiao had predicted that the new fee schedule would reduce the enormous disparity between procedure-based and "thinking"-based services. He had predicted that payments for invasive procedures would drop 42 percent, and that payments for evaluation and management services would rise by 56 percent. Now Hsiao was repudiating the basis on which he had made his earlier calculations. But this complicated scenario ran counter to the widespread belief that the health-care mess could be resolved—if only you cut physician salaries.

Not only was this story not covered, but high physician earnings continued to draw attention. One title ran "Doctors' Pay Underestimated but Resented Just the Same." It was a curious and misleading headline for the newspaper article that followed, although it did cater to prevailing audience sentiment. The body of the story compared what the public imagined executive health-care salaries to be with actual earnings. The public guessed what doctors, pharmaceutical executives, insurance executives, and hospital administrators earned. Then they stated what they *should* earn. People underestimated radiologists' and anesthesiologists' fees by roughly $130,000. They guessed $100,000, but the reality was closer to $230,000. But when it came to pharmaceutical executives, the public guessed they earned $600,000. This was shy by $1.3 million to more than $12 million. Estimates of insurance executives' pay were off by between $250,000 and $2 million. Despite the grosser disparity between fact and fiction in non-physician earnings, the headline focused all eyes on doctors.

A look at compensation in health-related industries reveals how paltry this nation's senior insurance executives would consider doctors' earnings—even the high-end ones. In his monthly newsletter, Joseph Belth, an emeritus professor of insurance at Indiana University, publishes a yearly list of insurance executive compensation. The 1992 lengthy list started in the $500,000s and peaked at over $12 million. (Unlike the medical profession, which now includes a high percentage of women, the list was overwhelmingly male, suggesting—as one male colleague did—that if you wanted to look for the really high-paid jobs, look where the women aren't.) The top rungs of health-care businesses remain overwhelmingly male and white—a story that also has had little press.

Distortions in media coverage come from a variety of biases, the most prominent of which is an emphasis on the "new" and the high-tech. These stories are covered at the expense of public health stories. Headlines cry out "novel," "untried," "first," "breakthrough," and "potential." Any sample of headlines from the best newspapers betrays the bias. "Scientists Report Novel Therapy for Brain Tumors" (a headline that made no mention of the fact that the technique was used in rodents, not humans), "New Device Set to Eliminate Kidney Stones," "New Test May Spot Metastasis of Cancer to Bones," "New Guards Against Infection." The significance of this "new" development is often moot or unexamined. Recurrently, stories are biased in favor of novelty rather than medical significance. Historical perspective is absent. While general news stories have their feet firmly planted in the present, medical news has one foot in the future. But anyone who has practiced medicine knows that today's advance is often abandoned tomorrow and that not all abandoned practices were harmless.

The novelty bias is exacerbated by a preference for success over failure—a bias that is equally prominent in medical publications. While headlines tout the advance, the text often carries modifiers like "possibly" or "still experimental," as though the limitations were less significant. Stories often bury the caveats and save the bad news for last. Variants on the theme include phrases such as "the study sample was too small to be statistically significant," "results are only preliminary," and a list of complications that is far removed in column inches from the optimistic lead paragraph. Failures of new technologies, even those that were yesterday's successes, are shielded from the light. When they fail, often they aren't considered newsworthy. But coverage of such failures might instill the public with a healthy dose of skepticism.

While the medical press suffers the same bias for success, its readership has learned to be more wary. Most doctors realize that today's breakthrough may have hidden complications, that its success is likely to be more modest than predicted. DES, a pill to prevent miscarriages, was found to cause cancer in daughters born to the women who used it. The large Bjork-Shiley heart valve was later found to break, causing death in two thirds of patients in whom it had fractured. The Dalkon Shield was a contraceptive that caused sterility. X-rays used to treat acne were later linked to development of thyroid cancer. Doctors' enthusiasm for the new is tempered by the responsibility for patient care, by the memory of advances gone awry. It is sobering to be the one to tell a patient that his heart valve must be replaced because it could kill him or to tell a young woman that she cannot have children because her contraceptive made her sterile. The responsibility of face-to-face care often makes one enthusiastic for the tried and true, rather than the new. One learns to trust the record. The history of medicine has a sobering effect.

While many of these "new" stories attract more attention than they deserve, the media lets "old" stories lie dormant. They are often public health stories which lack the glitz of new technology and the immediacy of human interest. They are often mired in eyes-glazing-over statistics, or complicated ideas that don't lend themselves to sound bites or visuals. The growing number of drug-resistant tuberculosis cases was one such story.

In October 1992, the *New York Times* ran a front-page story on TB, the first of a five-part series. Its subhead was telling: "Opportunities to Eradicate the Disease Were Lost." A resurgence of TB had paralleled the AIDS epidemic and the rise in homelessness. The development of a drug-resistant epidemic threatened to undo the progress of the last fifty years. TB would go from a curable to an incurable illness, the disease would no longer be preventable in healthy people who had been exposed, and treatment could cost a fortune. A case of TB that is resistant to multiple drugs can cost $250,000 and include prolonged hospitalization and possibly surgery. A case caused by drug-sensitive strains costs less than $1,000 and can easily be treated on an outpatient basis.

But this public health misstep wasn't news. It had been noted as early as 1990, seven years after the federal Centers for Disease Control and Prevention had stopped tracking drug-resistant TB. According to Dr. Dixie Snider, formerly head of the CDC's division of tuberculosis, a lack of funding was to blame. Not until 1992 did Congress have a line item for TB control at the national level. That was a curious decision given TB's link to health and social problems that were on the rise. Snider said that reaction was delayed largely because those affected lacked political clout. "What it took was for TB to affect AIDS patients who were backed by activist groups," he said. "The unions got involved when health-care workers and correctional officers were affected. Unfortunately, bad things had to happen first." The press, like Congress, had failed to recognize the threat of drug-resistant TB.

Public health issues also get drowned out by our love of high technology. A case in point is the story of the first baboon liver transplanted into a man. The story was front-page news, as was a teaser about the second such transplant six months later. Yet nowhere in the detailed account of the surgery, the immunosuppressive medications needed to prevent transplant rejection, and the plight of patients awaiting the limited supply of human organs was it mentioned that a preventable disease had destroyed this man's liver. He suffered from hepatitis B, a viral infection that is preventable by a series of three vaccines. Since the vaccine wasn't mentioned, neither were the obstacles to its widespread use, which include a lack of awareness that the vaccine exists and the vaccine's cost—more than $120 for the medication alone. There was also no mention of how someone contracts the virus—sexual contact, intravenous drug use, and maternal-to-infant transmission during birth are the most common routes now that blood transfusions are screened. The man's death, seventy days after he received the baboon liver, was reported in the newspaper's final section. The public health message had been lost: This man, after undergoing a $275,000 treatment, died because of a preventable disease. The heroics of our high-tech health care obliterated the failure of our system to deliver first-rate prevention services that include health education and vaccinations. The story reflected the bias of our health-care system generally, that high tech is more worthy than low tech.

Although the public health issues take far longer to capture the attention of the media, ultimately they have a greater impact on our lives, especially because we may get the disease or because we will pay when someone else does. Extensive play in the media could possibly alter the course of disease. An alert public is poised for health prevention and for pressuring the government to devote more money—just as it did with medical waste disposal. But public health stories play a distant second fiddle to the medical miracles of high technology. A striking illustration comes from coverage of two unrelated stories on one page of the *New York Times*. The lead, bylined, and illustrated story was "With Direct Injections, Gene Therapy Takes a Step Into a New Age." Its six columns surrounded and dwarfed a small story by a wire service titled "Teen-Agers and AIDS: The Risk Worsens."

An established science editor once explained that emphasis on novelty was justified because the media are not in the education business. That the media and education are inextricably linked, however, is made clear by Whittle's Channel One, a venture in which TV news programs are viewed in school classrooms. Students get the world news in exchange for watching commercials. Doctors, too, often get their information hot off the lay press. It's not so uncommon, when a significant medical story breaks on the front page of the *New York Times,* for doctors to arrive at the office with messages waiting from concerned patients wanting to know if the new development applies to them.

But the editor's remark begs the question. The media aren't in business to be didactic, but the educational side of the story may simply be background information that fits the news into context. Accuracy is a matter of perspective, not just fact. However, if people don't read the papers or watch the TV shows because they are bored, not only would they miss the stories, but the papers and TV shows would fold. If ads don't sell, if the show doesn't deliver its audience, then there is no TV, newspaper, or magazine. Medical news has to be able to draw an audience for the advertisers.

While some distortions of medical news are caused by the views of editors and reporters, others arise because of the sources they use. A staggering 90 percent of health stories are triggered by publicists, according to a public relations survey of 2,500 editors and reporters, higher even than the percentage of entertainment stories that begin with publicity drives. Press releases and video news releases for TV provide instant ideas and instant footage. Unlike advertising campaigns in which it is clear that someone is promoting a product, media coverage is couched in a guise of objectivity. Unfortunately (and for obvious reasons), reporters don't warn their audience that their story emanated from public relations firms, pharmaceutical companies, entrepreneurial physicians, or medical device companies. For reporters and editors under deadline, these press releases and VNRs offer quick, timely stories. The problem is that unless the reporter has a good command of the field and can put the story into perspective, the story can be closer to free advertising than true journalism. A gullible audience accepts as gospel what is actually promotional material, an unstated "advertorial." Shrinking media budgets, caused by the recession, help reinforce the trend. A reporter can fill more air time or column inches if much of the material is provided free of charge by someone else.

The former medical news reporter for CNN, Gary Schwitzer, described the effects of the "journalistic naïveté" of some of his television colleagues. "Most television medical reporting today doesn't help as much as it confuses, because it provides no context, follows no trends, and fosters unrealistic expectations on the part of the viewing audience." It promotes what he called the "gee-whiz" stories that delight publicists and alarm more sober, experienced minds. Schwitzer described the "educational" impact of such reporting on patients when he recounted the lament of a family physician who described requests for drugs and tests that were promoted on TV: "All of my best efforts can be undone in an instant by the education, free speech, advertising, free enterprise, and capitalism that are the American Way."

Despite criticism of some medical coverage, many reporters have done superb jobs. But investigative medical reporting remains scarce, often because newspapers or other media don't have the resources to let reporters dig. This is unfortunate, as the audience loses access to important stories as well as to an understanding of how things really work.

One of the most detailed examples of investigative press was coverage of the Dalkon Shield, a disastrous contraceptive. Morton Mintz, who first covered the story in the *Washington Post*, developed it into a book, *At Any Cost: Corporate Greed, Women, and the Dalkon Shield*. Mintz looked at the financial self-interest that led A.H. Robins, manufacturer of well-known products such as Robitussin and Chap Stick, to promote a contraceptive that would involuntarily sterilize thousands—even hundreds of thousands—of women and even kill some of them. Its insurer, Aetna Casualty & Surety, he reported, participated in the cover-up that kept the intrauterine device on the market more than a decade after its tragic effects were apparent. In 1990, the Justice Department abandoned a five-year criminal investigation into the case without explanation.

Another fine example of investigative reporting was a front-page *Wall Street Journal* story by Walter Bogdanich. He alerted the public to the fact that undertrained and overworked cytologists, paid by the number of slides they could read, were delivering faulty Pap smear readings. The Pulitzer Prize–winning story led to revisions of how cytologists worked and to new legislation regulating medical laboratories. Another *Wall Street Journal* story described how deceptive academic-sounding titles could mask public relations efforts. A group known as Americans for Medical

Progress launched an emotional attack on animal rights activists, with ads showing a white rat and under it the caption "Some People Just See a Rat. We See a Cure for Cancer." Without any digging, one might assume that it was the usual tug-of-war between scientists and animal rights activists. But the story disclosed that the group was basically a public relations front for U.S. Surgical, an $800-million-a-year company that manufactures instruments for the new techniques of minimally invasive, laparoscopic surgery. According to incorporation papers, the group was founded by four employees of U.S. Surgical, which relies on doctors learning their new skills by practicing on dogs. A cure for cancer wasn't the issue—selling medical supplies was. Similarly, the academic-sounding American Council on Science and Health appears as a press source to refute allegations of cancer risks from food additives. But corporate sponsors of that "council" include Ciba-Geigy, Dow Chemical, Pfizer, and Philip Morris.

In addition to distortions created by input from public relations sources, and a lack of time to develop stories, there are other hidden influences, like advertising dollars and corporate connections. Critics of the tobacco industry have attacked magazines for running too few stories on the dangers of tobacco, a lapse they attribute to the role of cigarette advertising. In 1991, the tobacco industry spent $264.4 million on magazine advertising—that was 4 percent of all magazine advertising income. The American Cancer Society ran a survey to see whether magazines would run blunt antismoking ads, testing reactions to several scripts. One unidentified publisher of a mass-market weekly objected to "More Americans die each year from illness related to smoking than from heroin, crack, homicides, accidents, fires and AIDS put together." Even though it's true. The American Cancer Society didn't anticipate similar objections from television or radio stations, since they are prohibited by law from running cigarette ads.

Behind-the-scenes connections play a hidden role that is hard to determine, unless reporters are also knowledgeable insiders. Morton Mintz raised the question of why the *Washington Post, New York Times,* and *Wall Street Journal* ran no editorials about the protracted suffering and legal battles caused by the Dalkon Shield. He suggested that corporate ties often steer coverage away from stories that are highly critical of major corporations. A veteran reporter at the *Washington Post* for nearly thirty years, Mintz pointed out that outside directors of newspapers were often corporate chiefs. He cited executives like James Burke, the former chairman and CEO of Johnson & Johnson, who was named as an outside director of the *Washington Post* at a time that his pharmaceutical firm came under fire for its own practices.

Coverage of health stories in the media, however, is not nearly as controversial as assessing the effect that TV and movie violence has on health. Researchers have linked TV violence to real-life violence, and violence is now finally recognized as a major public health threat. One study found that homicides among whites nearly doubled in both the United States and Canada ten to fifteen years after television was introduced—a period that was long enough for the first generation of TV children to grow up. A similar trend was observed in white South Africa, where television was not permitted until 1975. But a drop of 1 percent in the size of TV audiences would translate into a $250 million loss of advertising revenue. Although the ill effects of TV violence on children have been described since the late 1960s and despite the outcries over our current epidemic of shootings, violence continues to be shown and glamorized on TV. Bowing to the pressure of congressional outrage, the networks finally adopted a voluntary warning code in 1993. (But as a *New York Times* editorialist pointed out at the time, this was the same Congress that had refused to pass the Brady bill and had cut school antidrug programs. Although the Brady Bill subsequently passed, Congress has not acted quickly to curb firearms on the streets.)

Increasingly as reform has become a subject for medical reporters, I am struck by what seems a madonna-whore dichotomy. Stories tend to be polarized into doctor bashing and doctor worship, ignoring the more complicated, common, and ambiguous middle ground. Madonna status is reserved for two types of physicians: the superspecialists who perform heroics like transplanting baboon livers, and those who practice, Mother Teresa–like, with the poor. The whores include those involved in malpractice cases and those who overcharge. The dichotomy omits the vast majority of doctors who may not be deemed newsworthy but who provide the bulk of physician services.

In "Lessons on Empathy, Doctors Become Patients," a front-page story in the *New York Times* recounts "a national effort to train doctors to communicate with their patients," implying that the vast majority don't. The story draws no distinction between young students and more mature doctors, many of whom have already faced serious illness in themselves or family members.

The story ignores differences within the profession. It doesn't describe, for example, primary-care doctors who are sometimes left to mop up the emotional aftereffects of brusque technically oriented consultants. The story ignores hospital inhumanity that emanates from nondoctors, like transporters who don't talk to distressed patients lying on gurneys with nothing but a sheet between them and the great wide world. Ironically, at the end of the lengthy story on empathy was a brief fourteen-line unrelated piece about a thirty-two-year-old pediatrician with AIDS. Surely, he knew about empathy.

Another story, "Bedside Manners Improve as More Women Enter Medicine," opened by declaring that "as [Americans] lose patience with the gruff imperiousness displayed by many practicing physicians, some are beginning to suspect that the best guarantee against insufferable paternalism in a doctor is to make sure the doctor is a woman." In my experience, and that of my patients and friends, personality and specialty are far better predictors of imperiousness than gender. The imperious pediatrician is a rare specimen—whether a he or a she. On the other hand, complaints about female gynecologists are depressingly common. And the growing presence of women in medicine has not lowered the din of complaints or malpractice suits. In fact, dissatisfaction is greater today, even though the ratio of women doctors has increased to one in six from the one in sixteen that it was thirty years ago.

The media has certainly heightened public awareness of medicine. American patients are often well informed—not because they learn from their doctors, but because they read the press and watch television. But medical news also stimulates their appetite for new, expensive, high-technology procedures—at a time when health-care reformers are trying to trim costs. Americans, at least partly because of the media, are getting hungrier for health care.

CHAPTER 10

American Values—A Backdrop for Health Care and Its Reform

THE AMERICAN PATIENT has changed in tandem with changes in health care and society. The new turns of phrase—"health-care consumer" and even "client"—represent one of the most profound changes in health care, one that is leaving its imprint on health-care reform. Patients no longer trust doctors, even though they still make exceptions for their personal physicians. Once bound in a lifetime relationship, rooted in the community, doctor and patient are now more often in a transient relationship, one that nobody expects to endure.

Americans, boosted by self-help movements and patient advocacy programs, have seized a lot of control over health care, often from doctors who were distant or arrogant. But taking control of health care doesn't resolve the patient's problems of vulnerability during illness and of needing to rely on professional opinions. "Empowerment" can't fill a void left by a lack of trust. It is like a prenuptial agreement that offers protection if things turn sour but cannot substitute for a good marriage. We still need to trust our healers, because we are truly vulnerable during illness and because trust is part of the healing process.

Partly as a consequence of its disaffection with doctors, the public has tacitly given its consent to the remaking of medicine by business, the insurance industry, and government—institutions that are ruled by bottom lines and reelections. Public attitude toward physicians has helped remove doctors from the policy loop. In no other situation do people seem to believe that those with the most expertise should have so little influence over how that expertise is used.

Patients missed the distinction between trusting their doctors and having to endure a paternalistic this-is-best-for-you approach. Since patients must ultimately live with the consequences of medical decisions, they clearly need to understand their options and cast the deciding vote. But the decision process has to take place in a climate of trust, of cooperation. Too often now, it takes place in a vacuum of mistrust.

While Americans have grown increasingly sophisticated about diseases and their treatments, there is less understanding of policy issues. The public has given very mixed signals about even the most basic issues. Despite an apparent national consensus that health-care costs are growing too quickly, a recent survey by the Times Mirror Center for the People and the Press found that almost half the people surveyed thought that we spent too little money on health care. Only 7 percent of physicians surveyed felt that this was true.

While reformers harp on the issue of cost control, the public is more wary, seeing cost control as something that threatens their current access to health care, not as a step necessary to protect their future access. It's not clear that a lean system is what insured patients want—and they account for nearly 85 percent of the population. In fact, a recent study based on nearly thirty national surveys by major pollsters found a significant gap between public hopes and the recommendations of policy experts. The public doesn't want to lose their choice of doctors or their access to high-cost technology—over two-thirds even said that our country is spending too little on healthcare. Nor do they see high patient demand as a significant cause of spending. People seem to want cost control without spending—or getting—less.

Sentiment also can be easily swayed by public relations campaigns. Managed-care plans launched campaigns showing healthy children cavorting in bucolic meadows. HMO clients are led to believe that HMOs will keep them healthy (and—the subliminal message is—happy). But HMOs are often run by businessmen who usually assume no responsibility for patient care. The public seems to trust for-profit HMOs to put patient welfare above—or at least on a par—with the interests of shareholders and corporate officers. Only when people are personally burned by HMO policies do they seem to question whether corporate profits and health care are an appropriate mix.

Another indication of the nature of public trust and its sometimes facile sympathies was a survey of public attitudes to gene therapy. Done on behalf of the March of Dimes, the survey found that the public was overwhelmingly enthusiastic about gene therapy despite knowing little about it. Respondents thought that even employers and insurance companies had a right to know about someone's genetic defects—even though insurance companies then could refuse coverage for those who carry genetic diseases such as sickle cell or Huntington's disease, in all but eight states and employers might refuse employment. More than 40 percent endorsed the use of gene therapy to improve appearance and intelligence—not just to correct disease—despite the history of eugenics under the Nazis.

Other problems come from attitudes and expectations that are built into our national outlook. We have a great belief in absolutes, in seeing problems in black and white rather than in shades of gray. In the current debate on health-care reform, there is little mention of compromises or trade-offs. Changes are portrayed as purely beneficial, and the public remains remarkably unskeptical. While there may be a net benefit for most people and we may have no choice other than to compromise, nevertheless we would achieve a better solution if we saw the problems of reform as complex.

We also believe that doing something is better than doing nothing, a value that permeates medical practice as well. Ambiguities should be avoided, since they often signal a failure of resolve. The public expects to get better when they see a doctor—but that isn't always possible. Doctors, on their side, eschew the position that there is nothing to do. While many are accused of doing tests and procedures to make more money, even those doctors who work on salary share the bias that more is usually better. Doctors and patients tend to believe that medicine can always offer something. But this is only true in the sense that medicine can relieve pain and suffering, that death can be eased. Medicine may not be able to change the course of disease.

Unfortunately, people often want to leave no stone unturned. There is little understanding of the problem of "marginal benefits," of benefits that are too meager to pursue or too costly to justify. Patients are often reluctant to accept the ambiguity that "something" could be done but that it isn't worth doing. Instead, it is increasingly common for all the stops to be pulled all the time. This mechanized, no-holds-barred approach sidesteps the need for medical judgment. In our current medical climate, in which patients mistrust doctors and physicians fear malpractice suits, this course is often easier for both patients and doctors. Unfortunately, the cycle pushes costs upward and leaves everyone dissatisfied. A recent study found that the majority of primary-care doctors felt that patients sought too much care. Another study found that the difference in cost between the attitudes "when in doubt, do it" and "when in doubt, stop" could add up to $100 billion a year.

In addition to our tendency to view situations as absolutes, we believe that the best results are achieved by championing our self-interests. We don't believe that the greater good will protect our personal good, but rather that a greater good is achieved through competing individual interests. This tends to polarize us, to pit disease against disease, such as AIDS against breast cancer. Activists march under the banners of their diseases, believing—perhaps correctly—that they cannot rely on the kindness of strangers. Health care in the United States is fractious, as an unusual case illustrates. The birth of quadruplets to a poor, young mother prompted about twenty irate phone calls daily to the hospital where the babies were born. Callers wanted to know why a twenty-two-year-old had been treated with fertility drugs and what her million-dollar hospital bill would cost them in taxes and premiums. One person's care, or one group's disease, is seen to jeopardize others. "You get your care at my expense" is becoming our national view.

Our health care splinters us into interest groups. An initiative that would have helped the rural poor was scotched when veterans' groups lobbied against opening up two Veterans Administration hospitals in the South to nonveterans. The Senate squelched the project by a vote of 91 to 3 after intense lobbying by veterans' groups during an election year, even though the secretaries of both the Department of Veterans' Affairs and of Health and Human Services backed the pilot program. Our premium on individual rights and our emphasis of the differences between us is a far cry from the social beliefs that back the health systems of Europe, Canada, and Japan, in which more homogeneous societies band together for a common good. Sacrificing for a common good, in this country, is marked by the suspicion that we are being duped.

Without question, activist techniques work. The National Breast Cancer Coalition was instrumental in raising the National

Cancer Institute's spending on breast cancer from $197 million in 1993 to a requested $449 million in 1994. But there's a downside to our self-interest. Earmarking funds may stanch the basic research that yields unpredicted leads. And it can be a disincentive to limit costs. Filtering our medical expenses through the faceless intermediary of health insurance, we don't feel that medical care should have a price tag. One surgeon described a seventy-year-old man who was hospitalized for several months. The tab to Medicare (or the faceless taxpayer) was $275,000. Yet when the surgeon advised the patient to get a new pair of dentures so that he could regain his lost weight by eating, the patient balked—$75 of his own money was a lot. The money's source—not its quantity—set the perspective.

The Medicare Catastrophic Coverage Act, passed in 1988, was intended to solve a serious problem of the elderly—the potentially ruinous costs of catastrophic illness—as well as to add partial coverage of outpatient drugs and a few other benefits. But the elderly rejected this attempt to expand their benefits through their own payments. The Medicare Catastrophic Care Act of 1988 was repealed in 1989 because of their opposition.

Patients whose health insurance covers prescription costs sometimes ask their doctors to rewrite a prescription that calls for a single course of therapy. Instead they want a prescription for a longer course of treatment so that they only have to pay the copayment fee once. This behavior is far different from the patient who is glad to pay $60 rather than $120 for a prescription and hopes that one course will suffice.

We also believe that we are a classless society, that everyone is born with the potential to rise above the circumstances of his birth. We acknowledge that people can be disadvantaged because of race or sex but not that they encounter barriers based on class. Not only isn't that true, but the institutions that once mitigated the effects of class are faltering. Public education was once good enough to help people out of their economic situation. Blue-collar jobs were once paid well enough to lift the next generation into white-collar jobs. And the army, with forced conscription, was once a place to rub elbows with others who might offer better connections. But these equalizing forces are on the wane. Although we accept inequality in housing, education, and jobs, we pretend that this is unacceptable in medicine. We pretend that we can give everyone everything. Rather than trying to set realistic medical goals, we would rather pretend that only the best for everyone will do. We want Armani clothes to be sold at Gap prices.

Our legal system has also mired the public's medical options. If patients have gained control in the doctor's office, they have lost it in the legal system. Nowhere has this been more apparent than in right-to-die cases. Decisions that were once made privately, in the spoken and unspoken communication between doctors and patients, have been increasingly the subject of litigation. One of the most ironic and damaging cases involved a husband who tried to have his comatose wife's feeding tube disconnected after she was transferred to a nursing home.

The sixty-year-old woman had been hospitalized because of bleeding into her brain. Her condition deteriorated quickly, and one month later she was in a vegetative state. Her husband of thirty-six years consented to a special feeding tube so that his wife could be moved to a nursing home, but only after he was told that his refusal to do so would result in "legal proceedings." His wife had explicitly told him that she didn't want to be kept alive if there was no hope of recovery. Their two children and his wife's sister confirmed that these were her explicit wishes, voiced when a family friend had suffered a severe stroke.

One month after his wife's confinement in a nursing home, the husband asked that the feeding tube be removed. He was told—erroneously—that state law prohibited this. He was subsequently sent a bill for $18,500. The nursing home sued him for the money, and he sued to have the tube removed.

At trial, the judge refused to have the feedings discontinued, saying that the woman did not "contemplate death by starvation or dehydration." This was overturned by the appeals court. This appeals judge ruled that the provider was not entitled to reimbursement for services provided against the patient's wishes. The tube was removed and the patient died.

But that wasn't the end of the case. The nursing home appealed. A four-judge panel, by a vote of 3 to 1, ruled that the nursing home was entitled to payment for its unwanted services. The bill came to more than $100,000. Not only had the legal system wrested the medical decision from the family, but it had enforced the family's financial vulnerability as well.

Health care—and its reform—take place against the backdrop of our social values. We have always been an individualistic society, but today that characteristic is marked by more antagonism. We have long believed in science and technology as a means to a better future. But in medicine, we have discovered a dark side to this progress: the loss of human warmth and a high price tag. And we are a society uncomfortable with the notion of trade-offs. That is unfortunate, because we might do a better job with health-care reform if we made the trade-offs openly.

CHAPTER 11

Government

THE CLINTONS' DRIVE to reform health care, to guarantee security for all, may look like government is getting into the act for the first time, because we think of our fragmented system as private. But even before government set out to revamp health care, to create some form of unified system, we had a blend of public intervention and private initiative. Government already played an instrumental role in health care.

The federal government created Medicare and Medicaid, set tax policies which subsidized certain industries, influenced medical agendas at national institutes, and collected PAC money that sometimes guided their views. State governments played a role in shaping Medicaid at the local level, and several states seized the initiative on health reform when federal legislators failed. It was a hodgepodge of actions, but medicine ceased being a fully private, free-market endeavor decades ago.

When the federal government created Medicare and Medicaid in 1965, it stamped health care with a peculiarly American feature. It institutionalized a fragmented system. The old and the poor were officially pulled out of the common pot. Although removing these two high-risk groups might at first appear to bolster the private system by leaving the healthier behind, it set the stage for segregating patients. Health insurers followed government's lead, carving Americans into risk pools rather than distributing the risk.

Medicare, financed entirely by federal funds, insures roughly 31 million elderly and 3 million disabled persons (including 180,000 who suffer from kidney failure). In 1992, it cost $131 billion. Because of Medicare, the elderly are among the best-insured Americans—in fact, only 1 percent of those over sixty-five years old lack health insurance. But Congress has been less than fiscally responsible, uneager to antagonize its constituents. It has been loath to curb entitlements, although it has tried to rein in Medicare costs by freezing fees and to lower Medicaid costs by shifting payment obligations to state budgets.

If Medicare segregated one group of patients, it also compartmentalized benefits. Outpatient medications and long-term custodial care were excluded from coverage. This too became a pervasive feature of our health-care system. Where other countries have sought to manipulate copayments and to provide broader services, we have tried to exclude categories like dental care or preventive services. We have avoided looking at health care in a global context, fearful that it would unleash an insatiable appetite for benefits.

Medicaid, a joint venture between federal and state governments, was intended to provide health insurance for the poor. In 1992, Medicaid covered nearly 32 million people at a cost of $118 billion. But many, and in some communities most, of the poor fall through the net. Although low-income households make up 75 percent of Medicaid beneficiaries, they get only 30 percent of the funds. Instead, 70 percent of the money goes to institutional services for low-income elderly and the disabled. While the popular imagination sees poor single mothers and their children (a group that doesn't get much public sympathy) as the beneficiaries of Medicaid, they don't actually get the lion's share of Medicaid monies. In fact, less than half of those Americans who fell below the poverty level in 1992 were eligible for Medicaid. A family of three in Alabama would have been disqualified by earning $1,788. While the federal government bears much of the blame for setting unrealistic goals, states have sometimes diverted funds, occasionally using Medicaid money for general budget items, like building roads or running prisons.

Whatever the cause, the reality of Medicaid is that it falls far short of its image as an adequate insurer of indigent Americans. Many poor families earn too much to qualify but too little to pay for health care, lengthy application processes discourage many from applying, and extremely low reimbursement rates funnel patients into Medicaid mills where high volume compensates for low payments. When the uninsured poor get sick, their care is charity care.

The federal government has often turned a blind eye to significant issues that were not obvious to the public, although of serious consequence to them. Cutting reimbursement rates for

Medicare and Medicaid has meant that local governments and the privately insured bear the brunt of cost-shifting. At least two states added significant surcharges to hospital bills of private patients to compensate for revenue shortfalls. New Jersey added a 19 percent surcharge to cover the hospital care of the indigent uninsured, and New York tacked 5.5 percent to hospital bills to pay for care rendered to the uninsured. (At one point New York added 24 percent to hospital bills to raise $160 million for state hospitals and $90 million for the state's general revenue—suggesting that not all medical costs are purely medical.) Such policies, which Congress conveniently ignored, set up rate spirals for the privately insured, particularly for those who weren't members of large groups.

Congress has also swept the issues of Medicare's solvency and fairness under the carpet. Because of rising costs and declining revenue, Medicare's hospital fund could dry up by the year 2002, according to trustees of the social security system. Optimistic projections, assuming today's conditions, found that the fund would be solvent until 2009; pessimistic projections forecast insolvency by the year 2000. But the scenario was even worse than it sounded, the trustees found, because the fund was expected to run dry before a projected major demographic shift hit in the middle of the twenty-first century. This shift would mean that instead of four workers supporting each Medicare recipient through taxes on their wages, there would be only two. The generation now paying social security taxes, which generate a $96 billion annual surplus, might see it as bitterly ironic that, at this rate, Medicare won't be there when they are gray.

The regressive nature of the payroll taxes that supported Medicare—a fact well known in Congress—also made Medicare financing unfair. Medicare is supported by a 2.9 percent tax on wages, split between employer and employee, or paid entirely by the self-employed. The tax affects wages but not passive income—those who live off trust funds and investments are spared. And until the Clinton administration, there was a cap on wages subject to the tax, although the tax kicked in on the first dollar. In 1993, the Medicare tax stopped at $135,000 of earnings. If you earned $25,000, every dollar was taxed. If you earned $270,000, or twice the cap, every other dollar was taxed. The fact that Medicare Part B insurance policies were supported by general tax revenues further increased the burden on wage earners. Medicare recipients are entitled to buy supplemental insurance, which cost

$36.60 a month in 1993. The insurance, known as Medicare Part B, covers outpatient services, such as lab tests and office visits. But the real cost of this plan is much higher. General tax revenues actually pay for 75 percent of Part B costs.

Eligibility for Medicare also makes the system unfair. Generally, anyone who has worked for ten years or was married to someone who had, could get hospital insurance under Medicare without paying monthly premiums. Someone who worked from age twenty-one to thirty-one and then retired on a trust fund that pays $200,000 yearly doesn't pay a dime for hospital premiums when he hits sixty-five, even though he paid Medicare taxes for only ten years. Nor does his spouse. On the other hand, someone who had worked on an assembly line until age sixty-five would pay the Medicare payroll tax on every dollar he earned for exactly the same benefits. Some employees of state or local governments also don't pay their fair share, since they are exempted from paying Medicare taxes. By the time these government employees qualify for Medicare, it is estimated that they will have paid only 40 percent of the Medicare tax paid by people who worked continuously in the private sector.

But unfairness and fiscal problems aren't the only issues troubling Medicare and Medicaid. Like many government programs, the money flows out without adequate attention to detail. In fact, a provision of the original legislation which may seem arcane except to economic sophisticates shows both how the federal government let these programs become cash cows (like the defense industry) and how Congress failed to look at long-term implications of their legislation. Part of the original law, according to Bob Fuller, a credit analyst at Standard and Poor's, was a provision that allowed hospitals to pass through their depreciation and interest expenses. This might seem a bit of economic trivia except that the effects were profound. "This set hospitals on a binge of buying technology, of buying revenue-producing equipment," Fuller said. Not only did hospital expenses soar, but the medical equipment industry mushroomed. It is the sort of trivia that should remind us that when the federal government revamps health care, the minutiae we don't understand are likely to have effects that we will one day feel all too well.

Overseeing Medicare and the federal part of Medicaid is the Health Care Financing Agency, a division of the Health and Human Services agency, the umbrella department that also oversees social security, welfare, and the Food and Drug Administration—to name but a few programs. In 1992, HHS had a $550 billion budget, almost 37 percent of the federal government's entire budget. Medicare was the fourth-largest item in the federal budget after defense, social security, and interest payments on the national debt.

The sheer size of the department partly explained inefficiencies that were noted by the head of the General Accounting Office in a report that cited government agencies for being unable to control billions in wasted costs. Medicare and Medicaid combined were the fastest-growing portions of the federal budget. HCFA's plight was also aggravated by staffing cuts. As the agency's budget soared, its beneficiaries rose, and its programs grew, the Reagan administration cut its staff. Whereas there were 4,857 full-time-equivalent staff members in 1981, this dropped to 3,962 in 1991.

While Medicare's low administrative costs are sometimes hailed as a sign of its efficiency, the actual task of paying the 500 million medical claims filed annually is given to private insurers who act as intermediaries. The General Accounting Office found that HCFA failed to supervise these insurers, who were paying claims without looking at their accuracy.

One of the earliest beneficiaries of the claims-processing business was Ross Perot, who built his fortune at the birth of this industry. Within three years of Medicare's inception, his company, Electronic Data Systems, became a financial blockbuster. EDS got the contract for processing Medicare claims in Texas, claims that were administered by Texas Blue Cross (a company for which Perot worked part-time). Texas Blue Cross awarded the contract to EDS without competitive bidding. The company's pretax profits soared from roughly $26,000 in 1965, which was 3 percent of revenue, to roughly $2.4 million in 1968, which was 32 percent of revenue. That phenomenal growth of EDS won the adoration of Wall Street. When the company went public on September 12, 1968, the price of shares shot up to 150 times earnings.

Medicare also illustrates the government's lack of leadership in health prevention. It has shown the same bias toward high-tech, expensive care that pervades American medicine. While Medicare has been willing to provide almost unlimited funds for expensive (and often futile) high-tech medical care, it lagged terribly in subsidizing cost-effective preventive services for the elderly. In this, Medicare mirrored the policies of private insurers who have long argued that they provide insurance for illnesses, not health benefits.

One of the most glaring examples was Medicare's unwillingness to pay for flu shots until 1993, even though influenza is estimated to cause between 8,000 and 16,000 extra deaths a year among the elderly. Flu shots became a covered Medicare benefit only after a four-year congressionally mandated vaccine trial. Not only did the vaccine improve mortality statistics—and presumably the quality of life for those who would otherwise have gotten sick but not died—but the vaccine saved money in the Medicare trial.

As Medicare grew increasingly expensive, Congress sought to control costs by revamping payment methods for hospitals and doctors. In 1983, Congress altered the way in which hospitals were reimbursed for Medicare patients. Instead of paying for each service, the government implemented a system of preset fees based on roughly 500 diagnoses. The system is known as the diagnosis-related-groups, or DRG, system. Someone who is admitted with heart failure is coded one way, someone with a stroke a different way. For each code, the hospital is reimbursed a fixed sum, regardless of how long the patient remains hospitalized. As could have been predicted, a new industry blossomed—how to code hospital admissions for maximum revenue.

The second payment reform targeted physicians. The intent was two-pronged: to curb the growth in Medicare spending and to narrow the gap in fees between surgical services and cognitive ones. The resource-based relative value scale, or RBRVS, was introduced in 1992, but doctors doubted its fairness from the outset. The first year surgical fees went up more than three times the hike in cognitive fees. And the data that were plugged into the formula were so seriously flawed in some cases that it seemed almost laughable. Since the only nationwide real estate data available were based on residential rents from the Department of Housing and Urban Development, according to a HCFA researcher, commercial rents were not used. Nor were there any data on offices that were owned rather than rented. Because it was felt that rent control in New York would falsely lower New York City data, HCFA decided to use the highest cost data in the metropolitan area—which came from two suburban counties in New Jersey. New York City residents will be surprised to find out that HCFA allows the highest real estate component of RBRVS to doctors practicing in Queens, followed by the city's suburbs, followed by Manhattan. According to HCFA, doctors in Queens have higher real estate overhead than those on Park Avenue— which is absurd.

Not only were data flawed, but so were the ways they were used. When calculating fees, there was a "50 percent site of service reduction" if a doctor saw a patient in the hospital outpatient department instead of the office, according to an HCFA statistician. But a doctor who maintains a private office is probably still paying his office overhead while at the hospital. It's like saying you don't pay the rent or mortgage on your home when you travel for work.

In the spring of 1993, as the debate over health-care reform spread, the government talked of restricting physician fees to control costs. They cited physician incomes that averaged $160,000. At the same time, William Hsiao, the architect of RBRVS, wrote that the "misallocation of practice expenses in the Medicare fee schedule results in serious underpayment for medical services . . . which could dissuade those considering a career in medicine from entering the field. . . . If all payers reimbursed physicians at this level, the United States could not maintain a supply of highly competent physicians." While our legislators called for caps on physician fees, the academic researchers who had supplied their data argued that fees had been set without taking into account doctors' actual cost of doing business and that "it is clear that legislation is needed to correct these deficiencies."

The federal government's effect on health care is not limited to its two main insurance programs, however. It also has an indirect but profound effect through legislation that impinges on health care. Its tax policies have protected the insurance and pharmaceutical industries, and its ERISA legislation has guaranteed the sovereignty of self-insured companies in setting their health benefits. The unseen hand of Congress has strongly guided our private system for decades.

Tax policy has allowed businesses to deduct the full cost of health insurance for their employees. This lowered the incentive to restrict insurance costs. Since employees receive health insurance as tax-free compensation, they too have little incentive to curb insurance costs. During the debate about health-care reform, a group known as the Coalition to Preserve Health Benefits sprang up to preserve the untaxed status of health benefits. The preferred tax status of health insurance is a boon to the industry, for it mutes opposition to the high cost of insurance. After all, $3,000 in untaxed benefits is worth more than what $3,000 in taxable income could buy in health insurance.

The preferential tax treatment of employer-based health insurance is estimated to save $60 billion a year for those who benefit, according to the Commerce Department. But two academics who advised the Clintons on health reform put the value even higher. They estimated that the tax benefit of employer-paid insurance in 1993 was worth $92 billion. Curiously, the government decided that individuals, either self-employed or unemployed, could only deduct 25 percent of their health insurance premiums. Individuals were stuck using posttax dollars to buy coverage that was inferior to and more expensive than the insurance available to large groups. It is also curious that the government never looked at eliminating the tax-deductibility of health insurance as a way of financing health care for the uninsured.

The federal government also sets priorities in public health and medical research by controlling the budgets of national health organizations such as the Centers for Disease Control and Prevention, the Food and Drug Administration, and the National Institutes of Health. The NIH, for instance, gets about $9 billion annually in taxpayer revenue.

Where there is a distinct political agenda—either from the White House or Congress—politics can override medical science. The favored status of antiabortion groups during the Reagan –Bush years squelched federally funded research programs that would have used fetal tissue obtained from abortions. Despite the hope that research using fetal tissue would advance the treatment of incurable diseases such as Parkinson's disease, Alzheimer's, and diabetes, President Reagan's Secretary of Health and Human Services, Dr. Otis Bowen, issued a ban in March 1988, pending a medical and ethical review by a scientific board. The antiabortion lobby alleged that using tissue from aborted fetuses would encourage women to have abortions. In December 1988, two panels of experts advised that fetal tissue experiments should go ahead, that there was no evidence that they would promote abortions. But the ban remained. Four years later, Bowen said the ban had been a mistake and advised the government to lift it. But President Bush vetoed a bill that would have lifted the ban, even though the bill also authorized new research money for breast cancer and ovarian cancer as well as for an inquiry into scientific misconduct. Bush proposed that instead of collecting fetal tissue from abortions, the government should fund tissue banks that would harvest fetal tissue from miscarriages and ectopic pregnancies. The President decided this even though a lead investigator at the National Institutes of Health advised that such tissue was likely to be defective and couldn't be substituted, and another NIH official said that nobody but the right-to-lifers believed the estimates of how many fetuses would be available through these tissue banks. President Clinton reversed the policy.

Abortion was the underlying theme behind yet another confrontation between politics and science in which politics won. This controversy was over the use of an abortion pill. Trying to force the issue, a woman who was seven weeks pregnant entered the country with a personal supply of RU-486, the French abortion pill that offers an alternative to surgical abortions. Customs officials seized her pills. Even though individuals had been allowed to import medicines for their own use since 1988 (after pressure from AIDS activists), in 1989 the Food and Drug Administration banned the importation of RU-486. Her case quickly went to the Supreme Court, which then denied the woman's request to have the pills returned. It is ironic that the abortion pill was accepted in France, a Catholic country, and rejected in the United States, a country thought of as pluralistic. President Clinton aimed to reverse the stance on RU-486, but the French manufacturer, Roussel Uclaf, has remained leery of selling the drug here, out of fear that it would trigger a boycott of its other products.

If the political bent of the White House can skew health policy, so can behind-the-scenes lobbying efforts that in large part finance congressional elections. After the National Institutes of Health rejected a biotechnology company's request for large-scale human trials of its AIDS vaccine, the company turned to a politician-turned-lobbyist to press its case in Congress. Connecticut-based MicroGeneSys hired Russell Long, a former senator from Louisiana. Long reportedly approached Senators Sam Nunn of Georgia and John Warner of Virginia, who attached a rider to a $250 billion Pentagon spending bill that guaranteed $20 million in funding for a trial of the company's vaccine. A $6,600 fee to the former senator was translated into $20 million of taxpayer money that was allocated against the advice of the nation's top health agency. Subsequently, bowing to NIH recommendations that vaccines from several companies be tested side by side, the government asked those companies to donate their vaccines for a multiyear test. Only MicroGeneSys refused what was considered to be standard industry practice. MicroGeneSys finally agreed to donate a one-year supply of its vaccine, but only after assurances that its development partner, Wyeth-Ayerst, would pick up a $10 million tab. The biotech company and three legislators were not flying solo, however. A large pharmaceutical company, American Home Products, had a stake in the vaccine, and other lawmakers reportedly also intervened, among them Senators Daniel Inouye of Hawaii and Bennett Johnston of Louisiana.

It isn't surprising that health lobbyists exert such direct influence on our legislators, since they have contributed more than $60 million to congressional candidates over the past decade, according to a study by Common Cause. More than $43.2 million of this money went to 519 of the 534 legislators sitting in Congress in 1991. The cost of congressional races makes lobbyists integral to our political system. In 1992, candidates for the House and Senate spent $678 million to secure their jobs. This was a 52 percent increase over the cost two years earlier. Those who won a seat in Congress spent more than a half-million dollars each to do so. Those House incumbents who ran in tight races spent even more—nearly $800,000. Almost 40 percent of election money came from PACs.

The enormous profitability of the health-care industry coincided nicely with the increasing financial appetites in Washington. As the industry mushroomed, so did its lobbyists. While there were 117 health groups represented in Washington in 1979, the number had grown to 741 by 1992, including 212 political action committees. Members of Congress who have been active in reforming our health-care system have not recused themselves from taking PAC money from the industry on which they rule. This conflict of interest is largely shielded from the public's view. But it will no doubt leave its imprimatur on health-care reform. What's best for Congress may not be best for us.

As the battle for regulating health-care costs has heated up, PAC contributions have accelerated. During the first fifteen months of the 1992 election cycle, health and insurance PACs gave $9.6 million to congressional candidates—a 22 percent hike over the prior cycle. The jump was much higher than that seen in other industries. In the latest election cycle, Senator Tom Daschle, a Democrat on the Labor and Human Resources Committee, had received the most PAC money as of March 1992: more than $178,000. Representative Dan Rostenkowski, chairman of the Ways and Means Committee, was next in line with more than

$162,000, followed by Representative Richard Gephardt, House majority leader, who has drafted legislation to control health-care costs. Senator Harris Wofford, the Pennsylvania Democrat whose 1991 election put health-care reform on the national map, got $74,000 from health-care PACs. Some of these were not just industry trade groups but specific companies such as Manor Healthcare Corporation and Hospital Corporation of America. "Managed competition," the linchpin of some reform proposals, may in fact be managed by PAC money, not by free-market forces.

Looking at the past decade, Common Cause found that the single largest recipient of health-care PAC money between 1981 and 1991 was Representative Pete Stark, the California Democrat who heads the Ways and Means health panel. He has received almost $500,000, more than one third of which came from the health insurance industry. Other big recipients have been former senator Lloyd Bentsen, onetime Democratic chairman of the Senate Finance Committee, who was a favorite of the insurance industry, and Senator David Durenberger, ranking Republican on the Ways and Means Medicare subcommittee, who was a favorite of the hospital lobby.

As the current debate on health-care reform shapes up, it's worth knowing that the health-care industry has generally given more to Democrats than to Republicans—with the exception of the pharmaceutical industry, which gave more to Republicans, according to the Center for Responsive Politics, a nonpartisan research group. Interestingly, President Clinton's first attack on the health-care industry, in which he decried the cost of vaccines, targeted the pharmaceutical industry. And his endorsement of managed competition, in which the protective hand of government would assist Americans in buying insurance, has been seen by many critics as a way of safeguarding the insurance industry.

If PAC contributions are obscure to most of us, there exist even more arcane ways of assisting legislators. For those Congressmen who incur legal problems in the line of public service, donations can be given to their "legal expense trust funds." Senator Orrin Hatch was under investigation by the Senate Ethics Committee for helping a business associate get a loan from the Bank of Credit and Commerce International, a bank that was closed because of allegations of fraud. But Hatch, as a senior member of the Finance Committee, which also had jurisdiction over health-care reform, was valuable to the health-care industry, which contributed at least $9,500 to his legal defense fund.

And as important as PAC money has been, the hidden hand of "soft money" may be more important. PACs, which must register with the Federal Election Commission, can make limited donations. In 1993, corporate and labor union PACs could donate $5,000 per candidate per election, and individuals could donate $1,000—but counting primary and general elections, that really meant $10,000 and $2,000 per election cycle. But "soft money," given to the political party rather than to candidates, allowed individuals and corporations to give unlimited funds. The two major parties collected more than $83 million in 1991 and 1992 in soft money.

Lobbyists and businesses also exert discreet influence by holding out the prospect of lucrative employment opportunities. When government workers, especially those in the executive branch and staffers on Capitol Hill, leave public service for employment in the private sector, their prior work may be very well rewarded. Representative Bill Gradison, a Republican from Ohio, resigned from Congress, where he was the ranking member of the House Ways and Means Committee's health subcommittee, to become president of the Health Insurance Association of America. HIAA, the Washington-based trade group that represents the health insurance industry, had been squeezed by the move for insurance reform and the recent resignation of several large insurers who had been a source of millions of dollars in annual dues. Robert Patricelli, who founded Value Health, Inc., a company that performs a broad range of services including the evaluation of managed care, was a former Deputy Under Secretary of Health, Education and Welfare. In the company's 1991 annual report, he is photographed testifying before the House Ways and Means Committee. The circuit between business and government, which promises lucrative salaries after graduation from public service, reminds government employees that their actions could come back to haunt or help them financially.

The federal government also affects health care through mandates, issued either by Congress or federally supported agencies. What emerges is a pattern of quick to mandate and slow to evaluate, of appeasing public concerns rather than acting on their merits. Programs are set into motion without regard to cost—which often has not been realistically projected.

In 1986, Congress passed the Asbestos Hazard Emergency Response Act, which mandated that schools be inspected for asbestos, which might then be removed or contained. It was done without regard to cost or to the allocation of scarce school resources. Although different forms of asbestos pose different risks, Congress didn't differentiate. It was estimated that by 1993, the program had already cost $6 billion to remove or seal asbestos in 110,000 schools. It was a questionable use of funds, considering the immense needs of our schools and the fact that contained asbestos poses no risk. Dr. Lee Reichman, former president of the American Lung Association, called the program "a waste of money. It should have been spent on something more useful." In New York City the opening of public schools was delayed in the autumn of 1993 because of concern about remaining asbestos. Yet health experts said that the risk posed by starting classes on time was less than the chance of being killed by a bolt of lightning. The risk of an early death from passive smoking was put at 200 times the risk of dying early from asbestos exposure in schools—yet presumably this didn't cause smoking parents to quit.

Fraud, not just inefficiency, plays a part in making mandates costly and ineffective. New York City found out in 1993 that the company that had inspected schools for asbestos had fabricated data. That company had been paid more than $4 million by the city over a five-year period.

The story of medical waste, recounted earlier, is similar. When the Medical Waste Tracking Act became law, it was opposed by the National Institutes of Health and the Centers for Disease Control and Prevention. But even this opposition hasn't prompted follow-up studies to determine its usefulness and costs. The only real beneficiaries were the companies that dispose of medical waste. For everyone else, the cost of medical care simply went up. At one New York medical center, the cost of dealing with medical waste shot up from $106,000 in 1984 to $835,000 in 1989. The Act was a pilot program that applied to only four states and Puerto Rico. But if it were applied to all U.S. hospitals, this program would cost about $1.3 billion a year—roughly seven times what the federal government allotted for childhood vaccinations in 1991.

The same year that the medical waste law went into effect, so did one that regulated medical laboratories. The intent of the Clinical Laboratory Improvement Act was to guarantee laboratory standards. Since hospital and independent labs already met federal standards, CLIA's main impact was on laboratories in physician offices. The problem was the law's execution rather than its intent. Among other safeguards, CLIA called for twice-daily quality control testing—without evidence that this improved laboratory results. CLIA also mandated regular on-site inspections—to be financed by fees from registered labs. The on-site inspection fees were expected to run from $300 to $3,000. Registration fees ranged from $100 to $600 every two years. The effect of the law, if not its hidden agenda, was to close physician labs by creating administrative and financial hassles that were disproportionate to the small scale of most of these labs. In any case, the money would have to come from somewhere. Although there were problems with physician labs, such as overcharges and quality control issues, roughly five years later at least five of the country's largest commercial labs would find themselves under investigation for major Medicare and Medicaid fraud. Metpath, Metwest, and National Health Laboratories settled by refunding the government $150 million. No private doctor's lab could ever have overcharged the public on such a massive scale.

Less than a year after CLIA was enacted, another medical mandate took effect. Under orders from Congress, the Health Care Financing Administration imposed a pharmacy-based review of Medicaid prescriptions. The new rules required pharmacists to screen virtually all Medicaid prescriptions for drug interactions, ferret out duplications, and counsel patients about side effects. Although some people estimate that the new program will trim between $10 and $40 million off Medicaid's annual $935 million drug budget, others doubt the calculation. In any event, there won't be a net health-care savings, since the program is projected to cost pharmacists between $70 and $140 million and cost states as much as $15 million annually. One HCFA official said during a telephone interview that little was known about the cost impact of the program before it went into effect and that there was no good research on the cost-effectiveness of drug utilization review in general. The same official added that the evidence is "not terribly reliable" that there is a significant quality problem. One possible motive, he said, was that when the mandate passed in 1990, the goal was simply to trim the budget. And, he said, somebody had said that this would.

Federal agencies have also initiated costly programs on their own. In July 1992, the Occupational Safety and Health Administration imposed new rules to safeguard health-care employees against blood-borne infections, such as hepatitis B and AIDS. For the first time, doctors' and dentists' offices were included. The extensive new regulations mandate hepatitis vaccination of health-care employees, new laundry requirements for protective clothing, additional safeguards such as goggles, and educational programs for employees. While OSHA estimated that the new rules would add $821 million a year to health-care costs, many people forecast that the costs would run far higher. Roughly one year later, an OSHA spokesman said that the agency had not tracked actual expenditures nor was he aware of plans to do so—at OSHA or at any another agency. But for some people, the costly new rules were good news. Among other regulations, they mandate that protective clothes be washed on the premises or professionally cleaned, they could no longer be taken home. That led one owner of a laundry franchise to say this could translate into $5,000 to $10,000 a month for the average laundry, revenue that included a 70 percent profit.

Many people consider that the new OSHA rules are overly costly and burdensome. The New York State Medical Society summarized the nearly eighty new rules in a booklet that ran more than 350 pages. OSHA requires that, among other things, health-care employers must keep medical records on each employee for thirty years after the employee leaves.

Not only are the new rules complicated and, in some instances, of questionable value, but they also fail to protect many people who are at risk. Medical students, whose inexperience may put them in jeopardy, aren't covered because they aren't employees. Health-care workers who are consultants rather than employees are also unaffected by the rules. Employees of public hospitals are also not covered by federal OSHA (although they may be covered by state OSHAs), even though public hospitals often have the highest rates of hepatitis B and AIDS and thus put their employees at higher-than-average risk.

The cost impact of government regulation has been tremendous. Hospitals, which account for over 40 percent of health-care spending, have been especially hard hit by regulatory burdens. A study of Pennsylvania hospitals from 1983 to 1990 found that highly regulated departments, such as legal and government affairs, saw their costs surge by more than 80 percent, whereas departments with little regulatory burden saw costs rise by just 5 percent.

Congress has also shifted costs by unilateral decree. To reduce Medicare's share of the End Stage Renal Dialysis program, Congress increased the burden that private insurers must bear. By law, privately insured patients who are diagnosed as having end stage kidney disease must be covered for a set time period by their private insurer. In 1990, Congress extended this period from one year to eighteen months. Rather than face the difficult issue of taming the financial beast, it shifted an estimated $56 million in costs to the private sector. Coincidentally, the move was beneficial to the powerful renal lobby because reimbursement rates are higher under private insurers than under Medicare.

While the federal government doesn't seek to justify its own mandates with statistical follow-up studies, it does collect data intended to quantify medical outcomes. The government has been at the forefront of pushing for medical standards, even though some of these are based on assumptions that make them of questionable use. Acknowledging that some inferences may be simplistic, it nevertheless aims to use the data. In 1992, the Health Care Financing Administration released hospital mortality data for Medicare patients showing that more than a hundred hospitals had higher-than-expected mortality rates. Although a formula was meant to adjust data for complexity of cases, many hospitals complained that the results were unfair.

This could be merely self-serving. But some hospitals pointed out that a high percentage of their Medicare patients came from nursing homes. They were likely to be sicker than patients who were admitted from affluent retirement communities. Other hospitals complained that a high percentage of their Medicare patients were admitted from the emergency room. They were likely to be sicker than patients admitted for elective surgery. In most cases, the cited hospitals served poor communities. The most valid conclusion was probably that being poor is bad for your health, regardless of how old you are.

Although officials who released the data explained that the statistics weren't definitive, they did claim that the data raised red flags. Of interest, one hospital, St. Joseph's in Atlanta, had been picked by HCFA for a demonstration project to test the benefits of a packaged payment for coronary artery bypass surgery in a trial that began in 1991. It was one of seven hospitals chosen by a panel of experts because of the hospital's high quality. But one year later, when Medicare hospital mortality data were released for 1990, it turned out that the mortality for coronary bypass at St. Joseph's was 6.7 percent—exceeding the predicted mortality of 5.5 percent. According to a HCFA source, there were too many problems interpreting the data to mean what they might have been assumed to mean. The hospital's numbers weren't statistically significant. It could have happened by chance. Of more significance, he said, was that while the anticipated mortality for bypass in Atlanta was 4.8 percent, the actual mortality was 6.8 percent—although the total number of cases on which this was based was small. "I'd be more concerned about the city of Atlanta," he said. To the lay person, these data might raise a red flag about a certain hospital, but to the real expert they said nothing about the one hospital but raised questions about an entire city. Although similar Medicare hospital mortality data were collected in 1993, the administrator decided not to publish the results, the HCFA source said, because of the "misinformation generated by the earlier report."

The belief that numerical quantification can solve problems is shown in the new fee schedule that Congress enacted for physicians treating Medicare patients. Not satisfied that visits could be pegged as brief, intermediate, or extended, the commission advising Congress divided them according to complexity. But the new rules denied the reality of office practice, of making appointments. Doctors schedule patients for a fixed time that marks the average visit length, unless they know ahead of time that it will be short (like someone coming in for a flu shot) or long (like someone coming in for a complete exam). Someone who is scheduled for thirty minutes may not take a full thirty minutes. But this is offset by other patients who may be sicker or have disabilities, such as arthritis, that make a visit take longer. If a patient has crippling arthritis, a visit that should otherwise take only fifteen minutes could take thirty. Scheduling patients involves scheduling with enough slack to cope with unforeseen problems and with the multiple phone consultations that are part of most doctors' days. Since it is not yet customary for doctors to charge for phone time—as it is for lawyers and accountants—doctors have to keep enough leeway during the services for which they are paid.

If the federal government and its agencies have been meddlesome in some areas, they have been negligent in others, most notably in public health. Little has been done to promote anti-smoking campaigns, vaccinations, AIDS prevention, prevention of teenage pregnancy, and gun control, or to stem the rise in tuberculosis. Opportunities to intervene through aggressive health education drives have been squandered.

While more than forty states restricted smoking in public spaces, the White House failed to take a leadership role until 1993, when the Clintons made 1600 Pennsylvania Avenue smoke-free. In the United States, where about one quarter of the adult population smokes, there are roughly 430,000 tobacco-related deaths each

year. Smoking-related illnesses are said to cost us $65 billion a
year. Despite the huge threat to public health, the federal government failed to throw its weight behind a huge campaign. Nancy
Reagan launched her high-profile "Just Say No" to drugs campaign, but there was no analogous attack on cigarettes. The
reason most likely lies in the economic clout of cigarette makers.

In 1992, Philip Morris alone had a $1.6 billion operating profit
from cigarette sales in the United States and overseas. Cigarettes ·
help our trade deficit. Overseas sales are increasing, especially in
the Pacific Rim and Eastern Europe. And cigarettes are good for
domestic employment, in states such as California, North Carolina, New York, Virginia, and Texas. The prosperity of the
tobacco industry has also been shared with our political leaders.
In the 1992 election cycle, RJR Nabisco gave almost $300,000 to the
Democratic party and more than $400,000 to the Republican party,
according to two consumer groups, Public Citizen Health Research Group and the Advocacy Institute. In the 1992 presidential
campaign, a key Bush fund-raiser had ties to the industry, and a
Clinton campaign official was a lawyer who opposed smoke-free
restaurant laws in California, according to the consumer groups.
The Bush administration declined repeated requests from Dr.
Louis Sullivan, then Secretary of Health and Human Services, to
sign an executive order banning smoking in all federal buildings.
Until the current health-care reform debate, cigarette taxes got
little federal attention. But hiking cigarette taxes would be another way to lower the number of smokers. In Canada, tripling
cigarette taxes lowered the number of smokers by 40 percent in
less than a decade.

Cigarette smoking also offers a clear example of how public
health is tied to nonmedical factors over which government could
exert an indirect influence. The link is through education. A
study of men and women between the ages of twenty and twenty-
four showed that education and cigarette use were indirectly
proportional: the fewer years of schooling that you had, the more
likely that you smoked. Over 55 percent of men with fewer than
twelve years of education smoked. Only 16 percent of men with
more than thirteen years of education smoked. The correlation of
smoking and education held for women as well, and across racial
lines. The billions of dollars spent on inspecting schools for
asbestos would have been better spent teaching teenagers not to
smoke—or even motivating them to stay in school. Looking at
public health issues, our government has often failed to seek the

lower-cost and more successful solutions that can be achieved through education and housing. In doing so, the government ignores repeated lessons of public health. The great advances, even for infectious diseases such as tuberculosis, often occurred because living conditions improved.

If cigarettes show the country's passive acquiescence to a public health threat, the country's repeated opposition to gun control has made it a more active partner in promoting a major threat to the national health. Gun-linked violence is increasingly a public health issue, not just a concern of the courts. In the early 1990s, for the first time, guns killed more people in Texas than motor vehicle accidents. Firearms have become the eighth leading cause of death, claiming more than 37,000 lives in 1990. In the 1980s, guns killed more than three times the number of people who died of AIDS and more than five times the number of Americans who died in Vietnam. Deaths aren't the only cost. One study estimated that there are more than seven gun-related injuries for every gun-caused death. Another study found that in Detroit, bullets cause 40 percent of spinal cord injuries. In 1988, the health-care costs of firearm injuries were estimated to be $16.2 billion. Yet the gun lobby would have us believe that ownership is guaranteed by the Constitution and that it protects us in our homes. Instead, the 200 million guns in private hands have given us a national epidemic of violence protected by our government. At least one Congressman, John Dingell, is active in health legislation and in the National Rifle Association, of which he is a board member.

AIDS offers another glaring example of the government's failure to use public health aggressively to prevent illness and death. The federal government preferred to earmark dollars for research, an antiseptic approach that doesn't involve talking about sex, homosexuality, or drug abuse, especially in the detail that is needed to provide truly useful information. This prudishness has cost thousands of lives and shifted the emphasis from inexpensive and effective prevention to high-cost, high-tech, and—to what is for now—ineffectual treatment. Several European countries chose a decidedly different course. In Finland, the national Health Authority mailed a brochure to every sixteen-year-old that pictured a nude couple embracing. A latex condom and a message about safer sex was enclosed. The government also enclosed a letter for parents, about sexually transmitted diseases and abortions. Surveys conducted at Helsinki University found that 90 percent of those who received the brochures read them.

In Holland, a needle-exchange program was under way by 1985 in an attempt to slow the spread of AIDS among intravenous drug users. By 1992, 700,000 sterile needles were distributed in Amsterdam, a city that has 3,000 addicts. That same year, various communities in the United States managed to pass out roughly 2 million needles among the country's more than 1 million IV drug users. In Britain, by the mid-1980s, large urban billboards carried messages about AIDS.

The federal government has not only failed to take strong health initiatives—as it could have done with several public health problems—but it also blocked some state efforts. One of the boldest proposals came from Oregon. In an effort to extend Medicaid coverage so that more than 400,000 uninsured Oregonians might eventually have health insurance, the state ranked 709 medical procedures with a floating cut-off. Depending on the amount of money available, the cut-off would be made at varying levels. Treatments were ranked by a commission of doctors, nurses, social workers, consumers, and industry professionals. A waiver from the federal government would have allowed Oregon the flexibility needed to implement its Medicaid program. But after five years of state planning and public meetings, the Bush administration rejected the state's application for a Medicaid waiver, citing a possible violation of the Americans with Disabilities Act as an obstacle. Oregon's governor pointed out that she was unlikely to be insensitive to the needs of the disabled: One son was autistic and her husband used a motorized cart. Nonetheless, the Bush administration squelched the state's proposal, perhaps because the state financed abortions. Of interest, the plan's main author, Dr. John Kitzhaber, was both physician and politician—an emergency medicine doctor who was also president of the state senate. In stark contrast to many solutions devised by lawmakers without major input from health-care workers, this plan merged public interests and professional expertise.

Federal inaction also left states to devise their own solutions unrelated to Medicaid. Vermont launched an initiative aimed at providing universal health insurance by 1995. The 1992 law's only immediate action was to extend state-sponsored health insurance to all poor children. However, it laid the basic issues on the table with two years to come up with a final plan. The newly created Health Care Authority would consider a global health-care budget, aim to cut malpractice costs, and decide whether Vermont should become a self-insured single payer like Canada. The Authority would stress primary care over procedures. Interestingly, the plan was supported by the state's governor, who was also a physician.

While Oregon and Vermont tried to grapple with what to pay for—not just how to pay for it—other states tried to raise funds without dealing with policy issues. Minnesota planned to extend basic health insurance by taxing those who deliver medical care. A 1992 law stipulated that physicians, hospitals, and eventually HMOs would pay a gross revenue tax: 2 percent for doctors and hospitals beginning in 1992; 1 percent for HMOs starting in 1996. Minnesota doctors will also pay more for their licenses—$400 annually. Out-of-state doctors who treat more than twenty Minnesotans are required to pay the tax on these patients too. The legislators' argument for choosing to tax health-care providers rather than the public was that this wasn't a "tax" but rather a "recycling [of] dollars in the health care system." It was like taxing lawyers to pay for courts or teachers to pay for schools. As was the case with New Jersey's 19 percent hospital surcharge, legislators wanted extra funds for health care without incurring the wrath of higher-taxed constituents and without cutting any benefits. Whereas the sick were to fund the New Jersey plan, here it was those who cared for the sick funding the plan. But interestingly, labor unions in Minnesota also sought to have the program voided on the grounds that the plan violated ERISA, the federal law underlying self-insured health plans. They argued that higher prices would be passed along to them, thus violating ERISA, which guarantees that assets will be used only for those entitled to the benefits.

Government's record—particularly the federal government's—is important as we consider the promises of health-care reform. Enact now, pay later, has too often been the case. Since the high cost of health care is the single biggest problem, it is crucial that any new legislation take into account the worst case—not just best case—financial scenario.

It is also crucial that we devise a system in which science is not ruled by politics—whether that is the politics of PAC money, ideology, or even misguided public sentiment.

CHAPTER 12

Malpractice and the Legal System

EVEN BEFORE THE FIRST LADY—a lawyer—was appointed by the President—a lawyer—to head the task force on health-care reform, our medical system bore the growing stamp of our legal system. Whether it's defining death, deciding who is legally allowed to die, deciding that a patient's ailment is due to malpractice rather than disease, or ruling that specific technologies should be reimbursed by insurers, the law has played an ever-increasing role in medicine.

Courts have even superseded medical judgments of medical facts. One study found that while "the standards imposed by malpractice law usually derive from professional customs, state courts have at times imposed higher standards, requiring physicians to perform tests that medical standards do not mandate."

The most visible sign of the large role played by the courts was the rise of both the frequency and the monetary value of malpractice suits. Malpractice litigation has had several undesirable effects, which include pushing costs skyward, poorly compensating the majority of malpractice victims, and now targeting primary-care doctors who are supposed to become the backbone of the new health-care system.

From the mid-1970s to the mid-1980s, soaring awards caused a crisis in the availability and affordability of malpractice insurance. Doctors saw premiums jump by 50 to 100 percent from one year to the next, and sometimes by even more. Over a seven-year stretch, total physicians' malpractice insurance premiums nearly tripled from $2 billion in 1983 to $5.9 billion in 1990. Hospital malpractice costs more than doubled.

In the late 1980s, premium hikes stabilized. Whether this was the eye of a storm or its end remains to be seen, although trends in the early 1990s suggested that the lull was temporary. The average jury verdict had jumped to $1.7 million in 1990, an increase from a little more than $1 million the year before. Although most cases are settled out of court, higher jury awards are generally an incentive to sue.

The rise in malpractice cases is partly attributable to the growth of high-tech medicine. Diagnosis and treatment have become much more sophisticated because of advances in technology. Early detection of diseases like breast cancer is possible because of diagnostic tools like mammography. But the potential to diagnose leaves open the possible failure to diagnose, by misreading mammograms or by neglecting to order them.

Many new diagnostic and therapeutic technologies also carry an appreciable risk, even if complications are rare. And increasingly, many technologies are used to treat older and sicker patients, thus increasing the chances of complications. The Harvard Medical Practice Study, a review of more than 30,000 hospital cases, found that 4 percent of hospital admissions were complicated by an in-hospital injury. While most of these injuries were slight, 14 percent were fatal. Researchers concluded that "a major reason that today's care is so hazardous is that advances in medical science have made possible bolder interventions...often in more fragile patients." The stakes are simply higher.

Malpractice claims also grew because of financial incentives in the legal system. Personal injury awards skyrocketed. Contingency fees for lawyers, which are typically one third of the settlement but can climb to one-half for cases that go on to the appeal level, were justified on the grounds that victims couldn't otherwise afford to sue. But as awards mounted, they created ever greater incentives to sue. Malpractice awards, like all personal injury awards, grew because of higher payments for noneconomic losses, like "pain and suffering." Accident victims now receive almost half of their awards for this hard-to-quantify loss.

At the annual meetings of the Association of Trial Lawyers of America, lawyers swap information about growth areas in personal injury law. Hot medical topics at the 1993 meeting in San Francisco were reported to include injuries from penile implants and group B streptococcal infections during pregnancy. The association's outgoing president was quoted in the *Wall Street Journal* as saying that "health-care reform is our major concern at this point." Another past president strenuously opposed capping awards, saying that this was "not negotiable."

Yet one state's experiment with capping awards for non-economic damages suggests that the tactic does temper malpractice claims. In fact, this may be the only approach that has a proven track record to date. In 1975, California enacted the Medical Injury Compensation Recovery Act which limited pain-and-suffering awards to $250,000. That state avoided the mid-1980s malpractice crisis that swept much of the country. But if capping noneconomic damages is a way of dealing with the problem, that solution may be fading. In 1991, three state courts declared the practice unconstitutional.

While advocates of our current system praise its ability to compensate the injured and deter poor care, the reality is that the system is grossly inefficient. Evidence suggests the current malpractice system is unsuited for doing either, that its effects are both greater and weaker than generally assumed. Rather than providing fair compensation, it often resembles a lottery, a way of compensating some people for malpractice or the injustices of life, and leaving others to struggle with their injuries.

Despite assumptions that patients are litigious, studies show that victims of malpractice rarely sue. Looking at claims filed in New York in 1984, researchers concluded that less than 2 percent of medical negligence winds up as malpractice suits. Thus, injured patients are relatively unlikely to be compensated for negligence. On the other hand, research also shows that a "substantial majority" of the claims filed have nothing to do with "provider carelessness." Poor outcome rather than malpractice is often the cause of litigation, although most awards do go to those who are truly victims of malpractice.

The net effect is a gross mismatch between lawsuits and malpractice. In most suits, the doctor didn't commit malpractice. And, as already explained, most victims of malpractice are never compensated. Additionally, most of the money paid out to settle claims doesn't wind up in patients' pockets. Of every dollar paid out, fifty-five cents goes to legal costs. When patients do win a suit, they often have a long wait for the money. On average, claims against obstetricians and gynecologists take five years to resolve.

The incidence of suits is so high in some specialties that one would have to assume that the majority of doctors are incompetent if one felt the number of suits reflected true malpractice. At best, one might think that most physicians practiced poorly at least some of the time. According to a 1992 survey of its members, the American College of Obstetricians and Gynecologists found that nearly 80 percent of them had been sued at least once. The survey, which is run every two years, found a steep rise in the proportion of doctors who had been sued more than four times. In New York State, with one of the highest rates of malpractice suits, almost half of all OB-GYNs had been sued more than four times. By 1993, malpractice premiums for some New York obstetrician/gynecologists had risen to nearly $112,000 a year. Neurosurgeons paid even more.

Not only does malpractice insurance push up medical costs, but extreme variations in rates complicate setting standard fees. In 1993, a neurosurgeon in Chicago would have paid $191,000 annually, whereas a colleague in Minnesota would have paid $29,000. The same year, a general practitioner in Chicago would have paid $24,000 for insurance whereas his colleague in North Carolina would have spent $4,000 for a similar policy.

Malpractice costs also generate an inflationary spiral that reaches beyond the price of insurance being factored into fees. Doctors raise their rates to cover malpractice premiums, they order tests to document clinical impressions, and insurers raise their rates to cover the higher costs. Although the Congressional Budget Office dismissed the cost of malpractice premiums as less than 1 percent of health-care costs, one could easily argue that $9 billion could be better spent. Malpractice premiums in New York State alone topped $1 billion a year by 1988. To paraphrase a saying, "One billion here, one billion there. Soon you're talking about real money."

Added to the cost of malpractice insurance, which is passed along to patients, is the cost of defensive medicine, which is also passed along. Most doctors practice defensive medicine in varying degrees, ordering tests should the case arrive in court. Although the CBO report found that doctors would order many of these tests anyway, many doctors don't agree. X-rays may be ordered to document the absence of a fracture despite little clinical conviction that one exists—just in case the doctor winds up in court. After all, why should a physician try to hold down costs single-handedly only to put himself at risk?

The story of cesarean sections hints at the impact of defensive medicine, although, as often happens, it is hard to isolate cause and effect, since many causes often come into play. Our rate of caesarean sections is much higher than that of other Western countries. Coinciding with the growth of malpractice, C-section rates jumped from 4.5 per 100 births in 1965 to nearly one fourth of all deliveries in 1986. A study of more than 60,000 births in the mid-1980s in New York State found that rates of surgical births varied directly with the rate of malpractice claims in the region. The more claims filed, the more likely that a woman would be delivered by cesarean section, since C-sections allow obstetricians more control. The study didn't prove that the threat of litigation was the cause, but it was highly suggestive. Since surgical births are far more expensive than vaginal births, maternity costs went up. (The high C-section rate is encouraged by its greater profitability and convenience for obstetricians, but nevertheless malpractice threats probably play a significant role.)

One of the major effects of malpractice on medical practice isn't financial—it's the mistrust between physicians and patients, even when neither side has grounds for suspicion. It hangs like a pall over medical practice. For doctors, it undermines the nonremunerative rewards of medicine. For patients, it sabotages the therapeutic value of the laying on of hands. Sometimes it makes necessary care scarce. Because of the risk of litigation, many high-risk pregnant women have trouble finding obstetrical care. In fact, some communities have found that obstetricians are generally in short supply.

If malpractice premiums have been a burden for doctors and an ultimate cost for patients, they have become a profitable line of business for insurers and a source of revenue for at least one state. After a downturn in the early 1980s, the business of medical malpractice insurance became highly profitable in 1986. Profits averaged more than 20 percent of the premiums over seven years. In 1991, insurers had a 35 percent profit on malpractice premiums of more than $4 billion, according to the National Association of Insurance Commissioners.

In New York State, in the early 1980s, a malpractice insurance fund was created because doctors threatened to pull out of the state in response to growing suits and skyrocketing malpractice premiums. The fund was financed by a 5 percent tax on hospital bills, a cost that obviously would be passed on to patients through higher health insurance premiums and deductibles. Even though the malpractice crisis quieted down, the surcharge remained in effect. Over a six-year period, the fund took in $1 billion but paid out only $2 million in awards. Despite this, only $700 million remained. That meant that $298 million had vanished into the ether of the state's operating revenue.

A look at who is being sued and for what they are sued shows other disturbing trends. While surgeons were once prime targets when their operations ran into complications, primary-care doctors are replacing them as the most frequent targets. The shift reflects rising claims for the failure to diagnose illnesses. Looking at claims reported in 1990 and 1991, the nation's largest insurer for physician malpractice premiums found that the failure to diagnose accounted for over 35 percent of its claims payments. Surgical claims accounted for less than 22 percent of the claims paid out. Other insurers showed the same trend. If the country is looking to primary-care doctors to hold down costs, to stem the reliance on high technology, it will be counterproductive to make them practice more defensively. It is unlikely that they will want to shoulder the burden of controlling costs by limiting access to technology if by doing so, they expose themselves to greater risk.

As insurers, under the guise of managed care, make more decisions about health care, they have increased the burden of malpractice without shouldering the responsibility. Not only can a doctor be sued for his decisions, but—in effect—he can be sued for those of the insurer. A psychiatrist argued for a several-week psychiatric hospitalization for a twenty-five-year-old who was depressed and suffered from drug abuse. The utilization review firm approved eleven days. Soon after discharge, the patient committed suicide. Seven years after the man's death, the psychiatrist was sued. The psychiatrist was not found liable, but because of a legal issue: he was a cross-defendant. Both the plaintiff's and the defendants' lawyers said that jurors would have found him guilty if given the chance. Their position was that he shouldn't have given in to the UR firm's insistence that further hospitalization wasn't needed. He should have appealed the UR decision. While it is easy to say that the doctor makes the ultimate decision, that may not really be true. If an insurer refuses to pay for an expensive treatment, such as psychiatric admission or bone marrow transplantation, that treatment really isn't an option for most people.

The conflict between doctor and insurer, and its implications for malpractice, is growing. This is particularly true in nonstaff HMOs, where the HMO contracts with independent doctors but does not actually employ them. The HMO decides what services are covered—a de facto decision about health care. Physicians can be caught between recommending treatment that differs from what is covered and patients who don't want to incur or cannot afford noncovered costs. In staff-model HMOs, where doctors are employees, there is less room for shifting of ethical responsibility. Having the courts settle the dispute is unsatisfactory for both patients and insurers. A favorable decision may be issued too late to be useful—the patient may be dead by the time a verdict has been reached to pay for a treatment. Or a decision may obligate insurers to pay hundreds of thousands of dollars for futile care.

While most doctors worry about being sued for malpractice, some have found themselves sentenced to jail or community service for acts that seem to be poor practice, perhaps even malpractice, but not criminal. A New York doctor was sentenced to fifty-two weekends in jail after he mistook a nursing home patient's dialysis catheter for a feeding tube and failed to quickly transfer her to a hospital. An Indianapolis doctor was sentenced to 300 hours of community service for administering morphine to a dead man, something she said she did to control muscle spasms so his wife could enter the room immediately after his death. Although there certainly have been cases where negligence was so great that it crossed the border into criminal activity, neither of these cases would seem to have crossed the line. Yet the perception that malpractice suits are not sufficient to stem poor practice increasingly raises the prospect of doctors being threatened with criminal suits.

Courts have not only ruled on the quality of medical care but have also played a growing role in deciding issues of medical fact, whether it's to determine which services should be covered by insurance or what is the real injury—like whether an HIV-infected inmate who bites a prison guard should be charged with attempted murder. But they often do a poor job determining scientific fact, failing to grasp the nuances of medical science.

In ruling on whether a bone marrow transplant should be covered for an AIDS patient, one judge suggested that marrow transplantation for HIV infection was not experimental because the treatment was used for breast cancer. But transplant experts would be quick to point out that success with one disease doesn't translate to good results in another. When doing transplants for cancer, you have to eradicate the cancer with chemotherapy or radiation before putting back the bone marrow. The purpose of the bone marrow transplant is to allow high-dose chemotherapy which would otherwise kill the patient. In the case of HIV, there was no way to wipe out the viral infection from all cells, to eradicate the underlying disease before the marrow was returned.

Courts have also ruled against insurance companies that refused payment for experimental treatments. This a murky area, since insurers have often refused to reimburse patients for treatments that were not considered experimental by physicians, even though they were technically experimental. For instance, cancer specialists often use chemotherapy drugs for cancers other than those listed on the label as FDA-approved. Particularly if these drugs are expensive, as many are, insurance companies have refused payment.

But the courts have also ruled that insurers must pay for treatment deemed by the medical community to be ineffective and unsafe. A review of seventeen cases in which patients sued insurers for failure to pay for three dubious medical procedures—Laetrile, thermography, and immunoaugmentation—found that plaintiffs won fourteen of the cases. The review by researchers from the National Institute of Health's Office of Medical Application of Research came to some alarming conclusions. "We found that the judicial system seldom uses, and may avoid, published medical science," they wrote, continuing, "the system prefers live witnesses over learned medical texts, despite problems relating to qualifications or inherent conflicts of interest."

Recently, the courts backed a mother whose child was born with most of its brain missing but who wanted maximal treatment. The baby's care, paid for by her insurance company, involved a prolonged stay in the intensive care unit. The federal judge said that to deny ICU care for the infant, who had no chance of long-term survival, would violate the mother's constitutional right to raise children in the way she deems best.

In the area of medical risk from physical assaults, courts have ruled on the threat of herpes and AIDS. In 1988, a Connecticut judge decided in a pretrial ruling that AIDS was not a venereal disease, and therefore an accused sexual offender could not be ordered to submit to HIV testing. Connecticut penal code allowed for pretrial venereal disease testing of accused sex offenders. This was not an argument about the merits of testing accused sexual offenders for AIDS prior to conviction or about the value of testing rapists for AIDS. This was a ruling that AIDS was not a venereal disease, even though 70 percent of AIDS cases were sexually acquired at that time. The judge decided that "the diseases most commonly referred to as venereal diseases are transmitted almost exclusively through sexual contact—namely syphilis, gonorrhea. AIDS, on the other hand, is a viral disease; the manifestation of the HIV virus that impairs the immune system is transmitted in a number of ways." The decision flew in the face of medical reality. Hepatitis B and AIDS are viral diseases that are sexually transmitted. In fact, you could say that the deadliest sexually transmitted diseases are viral and that their main symptoms, unlike traditional venereal diseases like gonorrhea, have nothing to do with sex.

Courts also have taken a growing role because of the ethical dilemmas posed by technological advances. But this role has often stripped families of their privacy and of the right to make decisions which are intimately theirs.

In early 1992, a Florida judge barred parents of an infant born with most of her brain missing from donating the infant's organs for transplant. The baby was born without any cerebral cortex and thus had no chance of survival. The parents, who discovered in the eighth month of pregnancy that their child suffered from anencephaly, decided to continue the pregnancy in order to donate the baby's organs. But the judge's refusal to declare the baby brain-dead meant that the baby's organs could not be harvested until she died. By the time she died, at ten days, her organs had deteriorated too much to be used.

In 1993, A Missouri man's two-year battle to get permission to remove the feeding tube from his comatose twenty-three-year-old daughter finally ended. She had been in a vegetative state since a 1987 car accident. The case was reminiscent of Nancy Cruzan, a Missouri woman who spent eight years in a coma before being allowed to die. A New York case mentioned earlier added insult to injury: A state appeals court ruled that a family was obligated to pay for life support that it had opposed. The court ruled that a man was liable for the $100,000 nursing home bill incurred for unwanted treatment of his comatose wife. Not only was he emotionally vulnerable, but he was financially vulnerable as well.

The legal system has also impaired use of cost-benefit arguments. Since the existence of any risk is used to justify a legal claim, it is difficult to use the argument that money spent on one problem would be better spent on a different one. Lead, known to be potentially damaging to children, is now routinely screened for in young children. But in many settings the cost of routine screening does not seem justified by the level of lead-related problems in the community. The money might be better spent on something else.

However, legal action makes the cost-benefit argument difficult to uphold, since suits have been won and settlements reached based merely on the threat of harm. While that would be justifiable if there was a long time lag and no way to gauge current exposure—as is the case with asbestos—damages have been collected when harm was not likely to occur. A Boston lawyer won a $9,000 settlement for his client on the grounds that the landlord had caused the woman "emotional distress" by the lead paint in her apartment. The fact that the woman's toddler had a lead level of zero didn't alter the determination to sue. Thousands of lead lawsuits are pending, according to a newsletter devoted to lead litigation. The woman's lawyer was quoted in the *Wall Street Journal* as saying that "as asbestos litigation dries up, law firms geared up for toxic tort litigation are turning to lead." He remarked that "the floodgates are open" for litigation.

The irony that cannot escape anyone is that the nation's average intellectual standards don't seem to have gone up as lead has been removed from paint and gasoline. Overall, reading and math scores have gone down. Legal action is forcing diversion of resources to issues that correlate more closely with lawyers' fees than the health of the nation. Estimates of what a nationwide lead abatement program would cost start at $300 billion, since roughly 57 million houses would have to have lead paint removed. And, in reality, lead removal often causes children's lead levels to rise, because of lead-containing dust. In several Massachusetts communities (the state with the toughest laws), housing has been razed because landlords who couldn't get loans for lead abatement defaulted on their mortgages and banks didn't want to assume legal liability for the houses. Abandoned, these homes deteriorated beyond repair. Many landlords now won't rent to families with children under six, out of fear of becoming enmeshed in costly lead abatement programs or lawsuits.

As health-care reform develops, a new growth opportunity may loom. A former Justice Department trial attorney predicted that representing whistle-blowers in medicine will be a new growth industry as the nation tries to lower medical bills by fighting fraud. Since the Federal False Claims Act entitles whistle-blowers to 15 to 25 percent of the settlement, the winnings can be significant. A recent scandal in which several major labs agreed to refund over $150 million to government insurance programs netted the whistle-blower $21 million. That amount of money is too good not to chase.

PART THREE

WHAT TO DO

MORE THAN TWENTY YEARS AGO, Dr. Lawrence Weed, a professor of medicine at the University of Vermont, pioneered the "problem-oriented medical record." The new way of writing notes in the medical record became widely known as the SOAP note. It was an acronym for "subjective" (what the patient complained of), "objective" (what the doctor found on physical and laboratory exam), "assessment" (how the doctor interpreted the problem), and "plan" (how the doctor planned to diagnose and treat the malady.) The assessment part of the SOAP note included the differential diagnosis, a list of suspected illnesses causing each complaint, triaged in order of likelihood.

The SOAP note offered a structured way of thinking about each problem. It was like a filing system—you had to create topic headings and organize information accordingly. It put order into the random narrative of medical records. And it made records accessible to others who needed to use them.

For a patient who was depressed, diabetic, and had fractured his hip, each problem would get its own SOAP note. SOAP notes were easy for other people to use. The social worker and psychiatrist could follow the notes on depression, the dietician could home in on the diabetes, and the orthopedist could zero in on the broken hip. It was a way of making one's written thoughts intelligible to others who might need to use the chart.

For a known patient who came into the office complaining of a cough, a simple SOAP note might read:

S—52-year-old smoker complains of cough for the last two weeks. Has had fever and some blood in the sputum.
O—No fever. Throat is clear. Lungs show scattered wheezing.

A—Probable bronchitis. Must consider possibility of lung cancer due to smoking history.
P—Antibiotics for 10 days. Chest X-ray. Encourage smoking
cessation. Follow-up exam in two weeks.

Reforming our system is analogous to the SOAP note's assessment and plan. Part I of this book is analogous to the subjective
part of the SOAP note—the list of complaints. Part II is like the
objective portion—the exam. And Part III is a combined assessment and plan. Unlike detailed solutions that contain final line-
item budgets, I will emphasize the broad strokes of reform. It is
not a specific plan, such as recommending a single-payer system
or promoting the growth of managed competition. It is more a
look at the goals that should be integral to any system that is
finally adopted. It is a clinician's view of what makes the current
system falter.

While politicians and policy wonks have focused on specific
plans, many have ignored the realities of practice. Often they
seem indifferent. Health-care reformers have become so focused
on medical care that they ignore factors that ultimately may make
a bigger difference to people's health. To a clinician's eye, they
often miss the forest for the trees.

Some solutions have been disregarded as politically unfeasible.
But ignoring these issues is like rebuilding a house while dis-
regarding the engineer's report on the cracks in the supporting
slab. Where you put your efforts at reconstruction depends not
only on your budget but on how long you want to remain in the
house. If you hope to pass it on to your kids, the slab might look
more important than a coat of fresh paint. It you plan to sell next
year, unless you live in a state that forces you to disclose the
defect, you'll probably opt for the cosmetics.

Reforming health care is much more complex than writing a
SOAP note. It involves millions of people, millions of jobs, the
legal system, and it must be a plan that can carry us forward,
allowing for demographic and scientific changes. On the way,
some people will be hurt—jobs lost, benefits decreased, perhaps
entire industries undone. What is clear, however, is that our
current system is becoming too expensive and exclusionary, and
that without some intervention both problems are going to get
worse. We have to create something that is potentially stable, fair,
and flexible.

What follows is a generalist's view, a look at strategies rather than legislative details. Like a generalist who decides that a patient's skin ailment doesn't need a dermatologist but rather a rheumatologist (because the rash is a sign of lupus, not psoriasis), or who decides that a patient's racing heartbeat needs an endocrinologist to treat an overactive thyroid gland, not a cardiologist to treat a heart disorder, this is a look at where I think the problems lie. The generalist's job is to decide what's wrong, before calling in the specialists.

Reforming our current health-care system, however, is like being faced with a patient whose problems are so chronic and complicated that they seem overwhelming, like an elderly diabetic who can't see well enough to take proper medications and is depressed by ailing health and isolation. The skin ulcers and nerve damage make getting out and about difficult, worsening the isolation. The patient's children are consumed by their own problems, one son is an alcoholic and the daughter is the sole breadwinner for her family, now that her husband has lost his job. The home health care that the doctor arranged has been unreliable, and besides the patient is becoming paranoid and thinks that everyone is stealing from him. He wouldn't even let the latest person in the door, who happened to be the visiting nurse.

It's time to step back, to set some general goals. Tight control of this patient's blood sugar (the sine qua non of diabetic therapy) may not be the doctor's main objective, but a better emotional state might be. The physician also has to face reality—he has to deal with the community's resources, with what the patient's family can provide, with the patient's insurance status, his own time constraints, and a host of other variables.

If we're going to fix our health-care system, we need to set some general goals and some principles for getting them in place. It will be up to a variety of specialists—the economists, the legislators—to carry out the specifics. What follows here isn't a blueprint for reform, but it sketches the underlying principles. Just as there are many ways to be charitable or educated or athletic, there are many ways to achieve these ends. But reform plans that don't address these underlying problems will fail to achieve their aims.

CHAPTER 13

Principles of Reform

Level the Playing Field

Fragmenting the patient pool has allowed the twin issues of high costs and limited access to flourish. Rather than putting everyone together, thereby spreading the risk over the whole population and making us see these as issues facing everyone, we have carved Americans into multiple insurance niches. Insured or uninsured, the usual dichotomy, is a recurrent sound bite that offers little indication of the problem. The dichotomy suggests a relatively easy solution to the current morass: just insure the uninsured.

The problem is that we have accepted—and many groups are fighting to preserve—segmentation of the insurance market. Even the government's current proposals aim to keep it sacrosanct, although it pools those who are left out of entitlement programs. It's time to pool our risks into one pot.

Until the 1970s, community rating was common. People paid uniform premiums based on community averages. Since then, the insurance industry and businesses have carved subscribers into increasingly specific groups. Large companies pay rates based on their group's claims experience, whereas small employers pay rates based on individual employee health histories. While some businesses pay less than $2,000 to insure an employee, others pay more than $5,000. Small groups and individuals have found their rates going through the roof. Increasingly, they have become uninsured or underinsured. In response to the rate hikes, large companies opted out. They became self-insured and play by a different set of rules. Unless we're all in this together, long-term solutions are likely to elude us.

Interestingly, the city of Rochester, New York, is often cited as a community that successfully held down cost escalation and kept its citizens insured. Many factors no doubt contributed to this, but the city's insurance history is noteworthy. Testifying before Congress, Charles Bowsher, Comptroller General of the United States said that "one unique feature in Rochester appears to be the structure of its insurance industry. The Rochester insurance market has not followed the national trends we have observed toward fragmentation and segmentation." Bowsher went on to say that, like the city of Rochester, "the state with the lowest rate of uninsured, Hawaii, also has an insurance market dominated by two private insurers." Pooling everyone does two things: it keeps people insured and it holds down costs.

But the country has largely opted for salami-slicing its population. We have Medicare (for the elderly), Medicaid (for the poor), ERISA-backed benefits (for self-insured companies), 1,500 private insurers, CHAMPUS (the Civilian Health and Medical Program of the Uniformed Services for military families and retirees). We have insurance companies ruled by fifty states' differing insurance regulations, and we have self-insured companies that are exempt from state laws but subject to federal ERISA legislation. The result has been enormous variability in costs and benefits, unrelated to income or medical need. Depending on the insurer's clout, some sectors that don't carry their financial weight force others to carry more than their fair share. Privately insured individuals are increasingly made to compensate for the hard bargains driven by government, big business, and managed-care providers, who then cite their cost-cutting efforts as successful. Without looking at systemwide costs, who can really tell what is going on?

It isn't simply that our system embraces pluralism, a practice we hold dear. It is that we built this pluralism on unfair and deceptive turf. Pluralism should come from our options to choose the type of health care we want, whether that's an HMO or fee-for-service plan. Our pluralism is based on grossly unfair insurance ground that divides us. Lobbyists, employers, patients—almost everyone is fighting to preserve the inequities that have become our status quo.

Our tax codes, too, institutionalize inequalities. Employer-based health insurance is paid for with pretax dollars but the self-employed can deduct only 25 percent of their premiums. Employers don't pay payroll taxes on medical premiums, so it costs them less to provide benefits than income. While wage earners contribute to Medicare, those who live off passive incomes don't. And low-end wage earners paid the Medicare tax on every penny they earned, while until recently, high-end earners were spared the tax above a certain ceiling. Certain government employees are exempt from Medicare contributions, but they are still entitled to benefits when they reach age sixty-five.

Cost-shifting has made analysis difficult. While Medicare and HMOs cut their reimbursement rates to medical providers, these costs were shifted onto the unprotected backs of the private sector. Policy makers pointed to skyrocketing rates of traditional indemnity insurance plans, and attributed this to fee-for-service practice, which rewards providers for doing more. But there were other reasons. It wasn't just the providers and subscribers who were at fault. The explanation also lay in the nonsubscribers, the groups that had the muscle to drive their costs down selectively, shifting them onto the "full-paying" customer.

Medical costs are viewed as the responsibility of those using the system, not as society's burden. We wouldn't ask only those who have had fires to pay for the fire department or only those who have been crime victims to pay for the police department. But health care is different. Some states, like Minnesota, even proposed or enacted taxes on the gross receipts of health providers to pay for the uninsured. They didn't suggest similar taxes on lawyers to keep the courts going or taxes on schoolteachers to keep cash-strapped schools open. They rationalized the approach by saying that it recirculates medical dollars, thus preventing health care from absorbing even more money.

But that's a spurious argument. If society fails to control social ills, medicine can't be expected to absorb sicker patients without increased costs. If society wants unlimited technology, it has to be willing to pay for it. Society must decide how much medicine it wants, a decision that opponents decry as rationing. But ultimately, cost control is rationing. Society cannot simply open the faucet and expect providers to offer an unlimited torrent of services. We have to accept that providing a certain level of health care is a social good—an ethical obligation—not a commodity to be traded by special interests. To do this, if we are to do it fairly, health care has to be rationally distributed. Health care isn't a right, like free speech, but a service that for society's sake—both practical and moral—should be offered to all. Unlike rights, services are directly tied to dollars. We have to decide how much we want to spend, then spend it as rationally and fairly as possible. How much we spend is not the doctor's decision but society's. How best to spend it becomes an issue for medical experts.

The only equitable way to level the playing field is by income. Not payroll income but total income. Not age bracket or health status. And not by employer. It shouldn't matter whether you work for General Motors or for yourself, whether you work for the army or for your state government. Payment for health care should be based on the ability to pay.

This issue of fairness is central to any reform of health care. And it largely revolves around money. The young and the healthy, by definition, will pay for the care of the sick and the elderly. For those who think this is unfair, there is a hidden truth. All of us— if we are lucky—will one day be old. And most of us would rather remain healthy than need costly medical care. We don't *want* a bone marrow transplant or treatment in a burn unit. We just want to know that it would be available if we needed it, that top-notch and affordable care would be ours.

As a society, we must provide these services according to their actual medical need, not according to whether insurance reimbursement policies make them profitable. The number of rehabilitation centers, CAT scanners—whatever medical service is offered—must be based on society's need. We have to undo the insurance artifice and government incentives that lit a fire under several new industries, that made services available based on profitability rather than need. We should undo the pressure of public relations and advertising, often driven by lobbyists, that cultivates need when reality doesn't.

The most obvious way to make the system fair is to create an income-based system, unrelated to employment. There are different ways to do this, although we must avoid letting health-care revenue become part of general revenues. If we opted for a single-payer system, like Medicare, deductibles and premiums could be tied to income. This could be used to finance a variety of choices: fee-for-service, HMO, a mix of both. It puts us into one pot, with contributions based on the ability to pay. It eliminates job lock and the impression that health care is free, and it makes patients decide what amenities they want to pay for. Unfortunately, the most obvious solution may not be readily applicable to us. Our politicians seem to have decided that Americans won't tolerate a tax-based system, even if it is the fairest.

Maximize Choice, Minimize Third-party Intrusions

Most people don't feel trapped by their insurance policies until something goes wrong. Yet, anyone who has faced a serious illness knows that it is crucial to trust the quality of your health care. Assuring people that they can elect different health-care plans on a yearly basis begs the issue—people get sick unpredictably. If you get a brain tumor and feel uncomfortable about the surgeon assigned to you in a managed-care plan, it's unlikely that you'll want to wait nine months to change health plans.

Ironically, tax-based, single-payer systems like Medicare leave patients with the greatest degree of choice. Medicare patients don't have to choose from a network of participating doctors. Nor will their primary care doctor be forced to refer to specialists he doesn't know. Doctors working in countries with nationally-guaranteed health plans, like Britain, Germany, or Canada, may face greater restrictions on their billing practices, but they are far less burdened by bureaucrats and businessmen questioning their medical decisions.

"Demedicalize" Our Ills

One of the best ways to "demedicalize" health is by improving general socioeconomic status. People who are wealthier, better educated, and have better jobs are healthier—regardless of the health-care system. Several studies suggest that socioeconomic status is directly related to health, even after adjusting for specific health behaviors like smoking, drinking, and wearing seat belts. This even holds true for countries that have universal access to health care. The health differential between upper and lower classes in England actually worsened after the National Health Service was created, despite the new universal access.

But government strategies ignore this reality and are actually moving in the opposite direction. Health care takes up an increasing share of assistance to the poor. Medicaid now accounts for about 50 cents of every dollar that the federal government spends on the poor, up from 30 cents in 1981. Unless there is a steady rise in federal dollars, the expansion of medical costs occurs at the cost of education, housing, job training, and numerous other programs.

Some researchers have also found that, in developed countries, average life expectancy correlates with how egalitarian income distribution is. They found that best health results are achieved in industrialized societies that minimize the gap between rich and poor. It's a finding whose implication bodes ill for us. It's also an observation that goes unmentioned in the current health-care debate, perhaps because the one inequality that we perceive as acceptable—even desirable—is that of income.

Partly, our health-care system is so expensive because everything is treated as a medical problem. Health care has become a final common pathway for society's ills. As many as 70,000 elderly parents were dumped in emergency departments in 1991, left by grown children who were unable to cope, according to the American College of Emergency Physicians. The phenomenon is pervasive enough to have a name: "granny dumping." If it's of any comfort, we're not alone in turning to medicine to fix social problems. A large psychiatric hospital in the Guangdong province of China was reported to be overflowing with patients as citizens grew anxious about the stress of market reforms.

But we may be unusual in the degree to which we have accepted the breakdown of traditional buttresses against adversity. Where family, friends, and religious institutions once helped people pick up the pieces of their lives, the task has fallen to our medical facilities which are straining to cope with an aging population, growing social ills, and a breakdown in family networks.

A lot of attention has been given to the idea of preventive medicine, to routine care that may prevent more serious illness down the road. Some studies estimate that 70 percent of medical costs are due to preventable diseases. Smoking cessation, low-fat diets, and weight reduction could lower costs significantly. But these are preventive measures outside the medical arena, not ones based in the doctor's office.

Preventive services provided in the medical setting afford definite benefits for individuals, but they haven't generally been shown to save money. Prevention is better than cure, but politicians who promote it as cheaper are misleading us. Not only do screening programs cost money, but every screening method detects false positives, suggesting disease where none exists. If you find something wrong, you have to pursue it. While nobody disputes that Pap smears are individually an inexpensive test and that they help save lives, looking at aggregate data shows how much screening programs can cost. Performing Pap smears every year is estimated to cost nearly $2 million for every year of life gained. Treating a high cholesterol level in an otherwise healthy twenty-year-old with drugs is estimated to cost nearly $800,000 for each year of added life. What really cuts costs is shifting problems out of the health-care system whenever possible.

We need to target diseases that are primarily the end result of social problems left to fester until they become physical ailments. Anyone who has worked in urban emergency rooms can attest to homeless people coming in with infections, head wounds, and frostbite. The cure—and the cost cutting—is to prevent the underlying problems of homelessness and to provide shelter when that fails. We have tended to medicalize a host of other behavioral disturbances as well, finding the medical model more palatable. Wife-battering and substance abuse, for example, have been transformed into ailments.

We are quick to medicalize our social ills because of convictions that underlie our collective psyche. We are enamored of high-tech solutions, and these are what medicine offers. Smoking cessation got its biggest play when several pharmaceutical firms launched their nicotine patches. Little attention was paid to the fact that quitting cold turkey has the best long-term results. There is no magic bullet, chemical or otherwise. Smoking is a complicated addiction, only one part of which is a physical dependence on nicotine. Quitting cold turkey works better simply because it reflects the strongest drive to overcome the addiction. It's less the method than the degree of personal motivation that counts. A once-heavy smoker described kicking the habit many years ago. He said that he had fallen in love, that he had found someone he wanted to live for. People have different epiphanies, but transdermal nicotine delivery—the patch—is an unlikely substitute.

As a society, we have increasingly absolved people of personal responsibility. The driver blames the car crash on the person who served him liquor. It's based on legal theories of vicarious liability and comparative negligence, ones that conveniently shift liability to those with deeper pockets. We have embraced an it's-not-my-fault mentality. Whether it's a cigarette smoker blaming the tobacco company for lung cancer or a murderer blaming junk food for temporary insanity (the famous Twinkie defense), the idea of individual responsibility has grown unfashionable. We're living in "the new culture of victimization," as John Taylor wrote in *New York* magazine.

But a society cannot afford to absolve everyone of personal accountability, even as it tempers judgments with compassion. From a practical vantage, there simply aren't sufficient resources.

For instance, we estimate how many firefighters we need, but that presumes that we are not a society of arsonists. The calculation is predicated on an unspoken assumption that everyone does their best to avoid fires. Smoke alarms, hydrants, and fire extinguishers are for the control of sporadic fires that occur despite our best efforts. Arsonists exist, but if they weren't rare, our firefighting budget would soar.

To shift toward greater individual responsibility is not to let society off the hook. The end-stage, hallucinating alcoholic isn't suffering from a crisis of willpower. But, at the other end of the scale, a wife-batterer shouldn't be excused as someone suffering—by definition—from mental illness. There is a spectrum of destructive behavior, not all of which should be medicalized.

We have also turned our backs on aggressive public health drives, preferring to allocate health-care dollars to the treatment of individuals. Some of these public health drives would be aimed at medical problems that start with social behavior, like teen pregnancy or the spread of AIDS. We manage to launch advertising campaigns for products that promote hair growth and shrink prostates, but our national public health campaigns are sadly lacking. We seem less able to unleash our convictions without financial incentives as the driving force. We have also been stymied by moralistic views. We have chosen to let teens get pregnant and contract AIDS rather than distribute condoms in schools or speak frankly about homosexuality.

Eliminate Waste

If we're going to limit health-care costs, we have to curtail health care as a major grower of jobs. To do so, we have to simplify the system, trying to curtail nonessential jobs, like those in medical administration, which have mushroomed in recent years. When we consider different delivery systems, relative simplicity should be a major consideration. Managed competition, with its creation of regional alliances and a host of other new administrative units, seems unlikely to lessen administrative burdens. In fact, a diagram of managed competition drawn by a staffer at the Office of Management and Budget looked like the complicated pathways of an electronic circuit board. That complexity must translate into high administrative costs, as well as the potential for political battles.

When we look at specific delivery systems—like private practices based on fee-for-service in which providers are paid for each service, or HMOs based on capitation, where there's a monthly retainer fee for taking care of patients regardless of how much care they need—we have to consider the systemwide and long-term implications. Many HMOs show cost savings because of patient demographics and negotiated discounts, not because they are more efficient.

HMOs have touted their economic streamlining, but administrative costs of HMOs vary, not only based on the HMO but also on who's calculating. The quoted administrative overhead ranges from 2.5 percent to 19 percent. The academic literature does not support the industry's claims that it is necessarily more efficient than traditional indemnity insurance. One independent-practice-association HMO serving 110,000 subscribers was found to have 18 nurse reviewers, 5 physician reviewers, 8 provider recruiters, 15 salespeople, 27 service representatives, and roughly 100 clerks. The researchers concluded that this administrative staff was about equal to the number of doctors needed to care for this size community.

HMOs have also created new areas of waste, particularly the IPA type cited above. Many have imposed enormous administrative burdens on physicians' offices that they exclude from their calculations. Providers complain that they can spend twenty minutes on the phone waiting for authorizations for consults, but the providers' costs of doing business don't appear on the corporate bottom line. While policy experts decry the inefficiency of the solo practitioner, anyone who has worked in a large office can attest to new expenses. Computerizing offices—necessary for billing, collecting data, and other functions—isn't free. Somebody has to spend time inputting data, developing the software, maintaining the hardware. In the old days, a doctor only needed file cards. Competing HMOs also spend vast sums on marketing.

The HMOs that have best managed to eliminate waste are those with walls, those that centralize their operations under one roof. Although the quality of care may be excellent, these HMOs offer patients the least flexibility. There is a trade-off.

While it is generally accepted that a single-payer system would lower administrative costs significantly, Medicare may not be quite the shining example it is supposed to be. A letter published in the *New England Journal of Medicine*, from a Florida physician, pointed out that Medicare's low administrative costs were deceptive. Although the Health Care Financing Administration may have spent a low 2.1 percent on the administration of Medicare, that was just to transfer the money to each state's fiscal intermediary that then had the responsibility of distributing funds to providers and patients. In his state, he claimed, Blue Cross and Blue Shield spent nearly $8 billion to distribute $17 billion. Local administrative costs, he claimed, were greater than 30 percent. The Florida doctor is not alone in finding the reality of Medicare a far cry from its theoretical efficiency. On the other hand, not all researchers have found Medicare so inefficient. And it may be our best compromise if we want to guarantee flexibility as well as universal access.

While lowering administrative costs should be a top priority, there are other sources of waste in health care. Government regulations need to be correlated with science, not with unrealistic worries from the electorate. Educational efforts rather than costly medical legislation could be tried to calm voters' fears. Our lawmakers need to understand and accept the difference between low risk and no risk, and to limit their efforts to genuine risk. We are spending billions of dollars on programs that have little scientific merit—like the medical waste regulations, the school asbestos program, and many lead screening programs. We would do better preventing a host of social ills that ultimately surface as health problems—most notably poverty, violence, and declining educational standards.

Other legislative mandates that may have been well-intentioned have also been wasteful. Beginning in 1985, federal legislation required all emergency departments that participate in Medicare to evaluate and stabilize all patients who come through the door. If a patient complained of a cold, legally the staff was obligated to evaluate him. The General Accounting Office found that more than 40 percent of emergency department patients had nonurgent complaints. The biggest rise in ED use occurred among patients who had no insurance or insurance that doesn't pay the full cost of care, like Medicaid and Medicare. Rather than burden hospitals with costly mandates, Congress should have addressed the underlying access problem.

As we eliminate waste, we need to look at the potential hidden consequences. Remodeling the bloated health-care industry is like dismantling the defense industry. We need to preserve not only essential services, but maximum choice and incentives for high quality care. Many reformers are working on the assumption that managed care is the best way to do this. However, it may not be true, although it may be the best way to preserve the insurance industry. Other possibilities include a combination of private fee-for-service primary care with an income-related deductible and set, packaged prices for high-tech, expensive procedures like coronary bypass grafts and bone marrow transplants. We need to understand waste before we try to get rid of it.

Facile economic assumptions will undermine realistic solutions. The issue of hospital borrowing is a good example. If health spending drops (as is likely) and there's a drop in cash flow, hospitals that now sell bonds to raise money for capital expenditures may have to pay a higher price for their loans. Nonprofits—which borrowed $23 billion in tax-exempt bonds in 1992—would be the hardest hit. An extra 1 percent in interest rates would mean an extra $230 million in debt payment. Higher borrowing costs would either drive health-care costs up or dampen acquisition of the latest technology, according to Bob Fuller, the credit analyst at Standard and Poor's. After evaluating ten years of hospital cost-containment in New Jersey, Fuller found that long-term hospital costs rose as credit ratings dipped.

Since medicine is so fast-changing, we will have to become adept at minimizing seismic shifts in health-care industries without fossilizing health care or paying for unneeded services, since both are wasteful. We need better planning for the future. New technology rapidly changes the face of practice, as the growth of minimally invasive surgery shows. Whereas 16 percent of surgical procedures were done on an outpatient basis in the early 1980s, more than half were done in an outpatient setting ten years later. We will have to design the system so that it will remain flexible.

Separate Health Insurance From Employment

The link between health insurance and employment was an accident of history in this country, not a policy decision. If we're going to fix what ails the system, we should either sever the link or redefine its purpose.

Health care has to be looked at as a public good, not as a job perk. It is a service—like education—to be provided by a society that is compassionate, affluent, and mindful of its communal interests. We wouldn't make education conditional on parental employment, nor fire or police protection contingent on work status. Keeping people immunized against infectious diseases is hardly a personal luxury nor a benefit to be limited to the employed.

It would be possible to solve some of the problems of the current employment-insurance link by standardizing insurance policies, but to do so would redefine the role of employers who have reserved the right to determine health-care packages. Unlike countries such as Germany, which have employer-based systems that collect money from employees and employers for standardized health insurance, our employer-based system gives control of the package to the employer. After all, it is a benefit. In Germany, the employer is just the tax collector. Here, the employer is the arbiter of benefits.

U.S. employers have steadfastly opposed efforts to regulate their options, notably by objecting to modifications of ERISA, the federal legislation that gives them wide latitude in setting health benefits for their self-insured plans. Businesses, seeing health care as a cost to be controlled by them, have insisted on retaining the right to define benefit coverage. Self-insured companies haven't wanted to plug the gaps in ERISA because it would limit their room to modulate costs.

Employer-based health insurance in the United States has led to job-lock on a massive scale. People stayed at jobs simply because they worried that the illness they (or their family) had, wouldn't be covered if they changed jobs. According to a report by the Congressional Budget Office, business's claims (echoed by some government officials) that health insurance costs were reducing the competitiveness of American businesses were "largely overstated." Of greater economic impact for the United States, may have been the effect of employer-based health insurance on the labor market. Although this can't be put into numbers in the way that health-care costs as a function of a car's sticker price can be, tying health insurance to a job may prevent Americans from doing the jobs at which they would excel. This problem could be fixed by disallowing the exclusion of preexisting conditions and requiring insurance for everyone.

But another problem created by the insurance-employer link in the United States is that it often gives companies potential access to medical records. Employers don't just funnel monies, they oversee benefits as well. Although they won't get a copy of the medical record, employers are likely to know the diagnosis and cost of treatment. If the employer's premiums reflect the cost of a particular employee, there may be an incentive to cut costs by cutting the employee. This problem too can be fixed if we go to standardized benefits and community rating so that a sick worker doesn't cost his employer more than a healthy one would.

But that still leaves an administrative headache for business, especially for small businesses, household employers, and companies that rely on part-timers—those who can't simply turn the problem over to a benefits manager. When the employer picks up the lion's share of the tab, it also leaves an inflationary and false impression that health care is free, or at least cheap. Basing costs on payroll rather than income taxes disadvantages those who must earn a wage rather than live off passive income. And it is also a disincentive for employers to hire more workers. Somewhat cynically, one political economist explained that the reason to rely on payroll taxes rather than income taxes was that Americans tend not to pay their income taxes, whereas it's hard to escape payroll taxes. That assumption, however, seems a grossly unfair position on which to base health policy.

If the problems with our current employer-based medical insurance are really solved, it is unclear that business has any role to play in determining health benefits. Once that becomes true, there is little justification of the employment link, other than the habit of history.

Control Costs

Without cost control, health-care reform won't succeed. It's not that medical care costs too much, but that we are paying for it at the expense of other services like housing and education. Without some control of total costs, health care will become a black hole, absorbing society's energy without sufficient reward.

While the general focus of reform has been on competition, managed or otherwise, we might be better off building a system on cooperation rather than bidding wars. Competition generates its own waste and false promises. When Aetna Life and Casualty displaced Foundation Health Corporation as the health-care providers for the 800,000 military retirees and their dependents, the $3.5 billion five-year contract was 40 percent of Foundation's income, thus dealing a sizable blow to the smaller company. Perhaps an insurance giant like Aetna was better able to provide lower-cost quality care. But perhaps they were able to capture a market by temporarily lowering their profits—as the giant re-

tailer, Wal-Mart, has done. One losing competitor for the government contract complained that Aetna's bid would allow only
razor-thin profit margins. When the losing bidders petitioned the
General Accounting Office, the GAO took their side, recommending that the Department of Defense put the contract out to bid
again. Competition and the consolidation that goes with it, may
ultimately raise our costs and lower our options.

One of the most striking features when we look at foreign
health-care systems—regardless of whether they are nationalized
or private, fee-for-service or capitated—is the level of cooperation
that is integral to each one. Government, business, the medical
profession, and patients work together, to varying degrees. Although all the systems face their own cost pressures, they are at
least doing so in the face of near-universal access.

To the extent that we can cut costs voluntarily, we will all be
better off. Price controls have a history of backfiring. They become
a challenge to circumvent, and they breed resentment among
those who are selectively targeted. They do little to discourage
some of the behavior that drives prices up, and they may also
discourage advances that will one day improve health care.

Doctors could be encouraged to lower the demand for expensive
services, whether that's by training to prescribe less costly drugs
or to use technology more selectively. Since doctors generate about
75 percent of medical costs through their treatment decisions, this
is an effective place to look for cost-cutting.

Ongoing education of doctors about the cost-benefit ratios of
drugs is one place to start. Although drugs amount to only 5
percent of total health-care spending, some of the savings here
might be painless. Brand-name pharmaceuticals can easily cost
seven times the price of an equivalent generic. We could design a
system where insurance paid for the lowest-cost equivalent drug,
leaving patients free to pay the difference if they preferred to buy
the brand-name variety.

The medical community and government health agencies, such
as the Food and Drug Administration, could jointly launch
educational drives, looking at those drugs that cost a lot. In some
cases, physicians simply don't know how much these drugs cost
until an angry patient tells them. Combined academic and government sources could publish recommendations, citing where
lower-priced alternatives can be safely substituted. The sugges-
tion so often made, that a doctor prescribes a particular drug for

pharmaceutical gifts—like plastic pens bearing company logos or notepaper—is absurd. But the fast pace of new drugs entering the market does mean that doctors often learn about new medications from the companies that sell them. Each time a new antibiotic hits the market, doctors are bombarded by information touting its superiority. But the real benefits may be limited to specific situations rather than the broad indications for which these antibiotics are sometimes used. Doctors need more information that can be quickly absorbed. For instance, if a new antibiotic is launched, an advisory panel of medical experts could simultaneously release recommendations that spell out situations in which it offers improvement and those where an old generic is equally appropriate. A comparison of prices could accompany the release.

Doctors could be encouraged to use lower-priced drugs that may have minor drawbacks like needing twice-a-day rather than once-a-day dosing. Again, patients could be given the option of choosing to pay the differential if they preferred the convenience of the newer once-a-day pill, or doctors could request that the differential be waived where convenience made a medical difference. For instance, someone living alone who is confused and is visited once daily by a nurse would benefit from having once-daily medications that could be supervised.

But even a modest proposal like this needs the cooperation of other players. The public and the legal system would have to agree that marginal benefits may not be worth the cost. For instance, one clot-buster, t-PA, used to treat heart attack patients costs roughly $2,000 more than another, streptokinase. Is it worth spending an extra $2,000 to have a 1 percent better chance of living past 30 days? If 93 percent of patients treated with the cheaper drug survive, is it worth an extra $2,000 to increase the thirty-day survival to 94 percent? Obviously, to an individual patient this difference may be critical. But society will have to address these questions, to make some choices, if we are going to control medical costs.

Cost-benefit analyses can also be applied to new medical technologies. The principles are slightly different, though, because it ultimately includes restricting the application of technologies. Marginal value in terms of medications generally doesn't mean withholding a treatment, whereas it does with technology. Although some cost savings can be eked out by paying a set fee rather than relying on fee-for-service, major savings probably come only by reducing the number of procedures. One study found that 500,000 patients underwent bypass surgery or coronary angioplasty in 1992—for a cost greater than the total appropriations for the National Institutes of Health. The reviewers concluded that half of the patients undergoing bypass surgery did so inappropriately. While doctors' self-interest is seen as an obstacle to this sort of voluntary restraint, ignorance often plays a large role. The doctor ordering a test may not know what it costs or whether it is the most appropriate diagnostic or therapeutic tool. Rapidly changing medical technology, some of which offers minimal benefit at much higher cost, makes such guidelines necessary.

But as any clinician knows, a host of patient variables might persuade a doctor that the guidelines don't offer the best option for a specific situation. Price-oriented guidelines should remain flexible. A doctor may feel that the onetime expensive antibiotic is worth it in the setting of a VD clinic that caters to prostitutes, because these patients are unlikely to take a pill three times a day for one week. Or a doctor may feel that though a cardiac stress test will probably be normal, there is no other way to allay the anxiety of a forty-two-year-old man whose father dropped dead of a heart attack at the same age. Although questioning each decision is counterproductive, it might be worth talking to doctors who more often than not didn't comply with practice guidelines. This would be a far more helpful approach than justifying clinical decisions to utilization reviewers who guard their standards as proprietary and then wash their hands of medical liability. Psychologically, it is also more appealing, since guidelines are predictable, set by experts (as opposed to utilization review which can be done by anyone with a telephone), and cooperative rather than punitive. Instead of ferreting out doctors who deviate on isolated cases, the overseers could intervene when doctors recurrently disregard guidelines.

Another way to curb costs is by using motivation other than money. More health-care players have to be motivated by something other than (or in addition to) money. Even our national scientific institutions have emphasized money and commercial success, giving short shrift to the communal spirit of research. Looking at the giant human genome project, our National Institutes of Health sought to patent human genetic information well before there was any commercial application. It sought to do so on a wholesale scale, seeking patents for 2,300 genetic bits. Free interchange of information among U.S., European, and Japanese scientists drew to a screeching halt. James Watson, head of our genome project and codiscoverer of DNA's double helix, resigned. Britain's Royal Society condemned the NIH move. An English expert wrote that it would "be unfortunate if the reasonable expectation of commercial benefits disrupts international cooperation and sours relationships between scientists." The profit motive had broadsided pure science. It was a very American move.

It's obviously naive to think that money shouldn't matter. But people do have other motivations. To the extent that we destroy the pleasures of work—which for many doctors is their autonomy—we only increase the reliance on money. And to the extent we condone certain segments of health care earning as much as the market will bear, we lose our moral authority to ask that patients and doctors curtail their demands.

If voluntary reductions don't work, or fail to work quickly enough, we have to look for alternative ways to limit spending. Whether that's tying the rate of growth to the GNP or using global budgets or setting expenditure targets, the underlying economics will have to reflect medical reality. If we want unlimited technology for a population that is aging and being ravaged by social problems, that has to be reflected in the amount allocated for health care. To tie the health-care budget to the gross domestic budget without moderating the demand for services is unrealistic. It's like saying that you want a 4,000-square-foot house for the same price you paid for a 1,200-square-foot house. If you're paying, chances are you'll settle for less square footage than if you expect someone else to pay the bill. What society has to ensure is that basic health care is available and that, if possible, costs stay relatively stable with regard to income (something that hasn't happened in housing either). If we are to control spending, we will have to allocate care in a more open and rational way. Rather than looking at "rationing" as denying somebody his right, we may have to view rationing as providing everybody his due.

To control costs, we will also have to undo the gross disparity between procedure-oriented medicine and "thinking" medicine, a disparity that helped spawn the inflationary use of medical technology. While a certain differential might be justified on the basis of added years of training, greater risk assumed, or the cost of equipment, the current differential is unjustified by anything within the medical world other than habit. This massive problem is primarily the result of insurance policies, both private and governmental.

To lower health-care costs we will also have to enlist public cooperation. Medical care isn't free, although the costs can be hidden, shifted onto others, or leveraged for future generations to pay. In fact, many countries that finance care through payroll taxes do so at a relatively great expense. In Germany, for instance, the combined employer-employee contribution can top 16 percent of gross wages. To limit spending, both individuals and society must realize what health care costs. Patients understand this through out-of-pocket costs like deductibles and copayments. Society understands it through taxes.

Individuals are more likely to limit their expenses when they pay out of pocket, but the downside is that it has the potential to deter people from seeking necessary care. Some countries, like Canada and Britain, generally provide first-dollar coverage, although both countries have had to increase out-of-pocket costs and trim services to deal with rising costs and recession-strained financing. In systems that severely limit out-of-pocket costs, waiting times generally act as the brakes on medical services. If it takes you two weeks to get an appointment for a nonemergency complaint, the problem may disappear by then or you may decide not to make appointments for minor ailments. While the long waits in both the Canadian and English systems have gotten a lot of press, many dispute the impact of these restrictions. However, waiting times may be a trickier way to lessen consumer demand in this country because of our litigious inclinations. One possible solution is to offer people the choice of fee-for-service with out-of-pocket costs tied to their income or HMOs without such costs.

Society is made aware of its expenses through taxes. Any effort to finance medical care this way should have a dedicated tax—so it is perfectly clear how much we're spending on health care. We, unlike many of our European counterparts, are very reluctant to finance health care through higher taxes. We mistrust our government to enact a fair tax, and we are even more skeptical that revenues would be spent prudently. Tax money seems to vanish like expense account money—without worry. People spending their own money tend to make more frugal decisions. Other countries either have more efficient governments or, at least, their citizens believe that they do.

Move to Community-Based Primary Care

When politicians talk of access, they talk about providing universal health insurance, which is the major determinant of access. The uninsured (or underinsured) tend to delay necessary care and use emergency rooms for nonurgent care. Both approaches are less satisfactory and more expensive. As more people fell into the void of uninsurance, reliance on emergency departments grew. Between 1985 and 1990, caseloads increased dramatically, reaching 99 million visits annually, according to a report by the General Accounting Office. Ill designed to be the primary source of health care, EDs nevertheless became de facto local health clinics.

But although health insurance improves access, it's no guarantee. Reformers who ignore the difference fail to understand several major problems of access. Looking at Healthy Start, a Massachusetts plan that provided insurance to poor, uninsured pregnant women, researchers found that adding insurance increased the rate of cesarean sections without improving maternal health. Access to medical technology went up, but health status didn't improve. Those who assume that insurance through managed care guarantees better access than traditional fee-for-service insurance are also wrong. A Philadelphia program started in 1986 known as HealthPASS, in which Medicaid patients were switched into HMOs, found that many pregnant women did not seek early prenatal care, even with outreach programs that supplemented their HMO care.

Varied reasons account for the discrepancy between health insurance and access to health care. In some cultures, public assistance is frowned on. These patients won't use Medicaid even if it's available. Sometimes there's a language barrier; sometimes patients fear moral condemnation from health-care providers. Or daily schedules don't mesh with the hours during which health care is available. People may have jobs that make nine-to-five doctors' offices or medical clinics inaccessible. They might rely on the emergency department because it's the only service that doesn't require taking time off work, even if they are fully insured. In the Philadelphia HealthPASS program, many Medicaid parents and guardians failed to schedule preventive services for their children, like vaccinations or vision tests, because of transportation or child-care problems. Over 50 percent of HealthPASS patients failed to keep their appointments. Clearly, insurance wasn't the issue.

In communities in which lifestyle factors or geographic location play major roles in creating health problems, community-based clinics offer a way of identifying situations earlier and offering coordinated backup. Illnesses exist within contexts, contexts that both induce disease and affect treatment. New medical problems sometimes aren't recognized until a pattern emerges. The beginning of the AIDS epidemic, black lung disease, new street drugs, a fatal respiratory illness caused by the hantavirus that first appeared among Navajo Indians—such new health problems are easiest to spot when the concentration is high enough to attract notice. And they are most effectively treated when health providers know the community they serve.

Understanding the specifics of a community also offers the possibility of targeted, cost-efficient care. A study of more than 5,000 poor children in Orange County, California, revealed that lead poisoning wasn't a pervasive problem. Despite state-mandated screening of all young children in the program, only 371 had elevated lead levels—only 6 of whom were in the danger zone. All 6 were Hispanic and had specific risk factors, like living in a household that used lead-containing Mexican folk remedies or eating from unglazed Mexican pottery. Knowing this sort of information could help move us away from inefficient mandates, turning the money toward better use in the community.

But it isn't just physical ailments that lend themselves to community-based health care. Deficient housing, education, or employment also ravages communities, often drawing limited notice as sporadic complaints of stress, alcoholism, or depression. Since these can be community-wide ills, they would benefit from comprehensive programs targeted at the broader problems rather than their medical manifestations.

Local clinics offer a way of integrating occupational and environmental medicine with care on the individual level. Farming, hunting, driving trucks—many occupations and recreational activities have been linked to specific health problems. A study of San Francisco bus drivers suffering from hypertension found that 60 percent were either untreated or poorly treated, despite access to medical care. Looking at the situation more closely showed that many drivers had been given diuretics (water pills) but couldn't use them. Even though the treatment was cheap and required only one pill a day, drivers didn't have access to bathrooms on their tightly scheduled routes. Community-based clinics also offer the benefit of easier physical access—a particular bonus in dealing with elderly patients, young children, or poorly motivated patients. School clinics can tend to students in their own environment, work-site clinics to employees. Neither involves taking time off, and both understand the intricacies of their environment. They can serve several purposes simultaneously, offering health promotion programs like smoking cessation, providing treatment of routine illnesses like hypertension, and arranging for specialty consultations.

Community-based clinics are well positioned to bridge the gaps between general primary care, public health policies, and sophisticated specialty care. Because clinic staff understand specific population needs, they can devise innovative programs. A test program that enlisted school and parental support was able to reduce emergency department use while offering kids better access to care. Some schools joined the state pilot programs in which uninsured kids were enrolled in insurance plans. Preliminary results from one Florida plan found a 35 percent drop in emergency department visits by low-income children after the local school-based program started.

One possible solution to our fragmented and costly system is to encourage enrollment in community-based HMOs, like Kaiser Permanente, Health Insurance Plan of Greater New York, the Harvard Community Health Plan, or the Group Health Cooperative of Puget Sound. These HMOs with walls would be the health equivalent of public schools. They could be run by HMOs with successful track records. Whether these are nonprofit or for-profit HMOs seems to make little difference, since profit status has become mainly a distinction of tax status, according to Dr. John Ludden, corporate medical director of the nonprofit Harvard Community Health Plan. But other alternatives exist. Outpatient facilities could be attached to local hospitals (to be staffed by fully trained doctors rather than doctors-in-training). The key to making the HMO with walls the mainstay of American health care would be the ability to draw the lion's share of middle-class patients, in the same way that most middle-class children go to public schools.

But this isn't the only possible system—and it may not be the one most Americans want. We could expand Medicare for all with copayments that are large enough to discourage excessive use and premiums that reflect real costs. Providers and patients in the Medicare model would live with negotiated fees. People who wanted private medical care—and providers who wanted to remain outside any system—would rely on private insurance.

While critics of this idea—a multitier system with HMOs acting as the lowest-priced option for universal coverage—might derisively cite the quality of public education in this country, it is unlikely that even they would propose doing away with public schools. Even many who send their children to private school appreciate the security of having the public school system to fall back on if their financial position were to change. And as a society, we would all suffer without minimal educational goals for all our population. The same could be said of health care. Well-run HMOs with walls, or hospital-based equivalents—designed to draw in the middle class rather than to repel anyone who could possibly afford better—might offer us one solution.

Those who prefer the more personal setting of their private doctor's office and those who want to pay for the freedom of fee-for-service could opt for higher premiums to pay for "Medicare" as well as higher copayments. This level of care, also funded by tax revenue, would have certain restrictions, like maximum allowable charges for specific services. Those who wanted additional coverage to guarantee maximal freedom, and to use health providers unwilling to abide by fee structures, could buy supplemental insurance policies.

The impetus to use HMOs would be that HMOs offered care with the least out-of-pocket costs. HMOs would provide peace of mind and comprehensive benefits, the twin goals of nationally guaranteed health care. People who wanted the next tier of service could pay more for a system like Medicare. Standardized, supplemental insurance policies—like Medigap policies—could be available for additional coverage. Just as taxpayers fund public schools whether or not they use them, we would pay for universal publicly assisted coverage even if we chose to buy our way out of it. People at the top would be buying a higher level of freedom and better amenities. But that exists already. If you want a private room or private duty nursing, you pay for it. On the other hand, you get the same operating room staff either way.

Lessons from Abroad

American medicine prides itself on being the best in the world. Yet Americans are not very satisfied. We feel insecure about the costs and the capriciousness of our health insurance, and often we feel as though medicine—a highly personal matter—has become dehumanized. We may be satisfied in retrospect with the care we get, but looking ahead, we are often afraid. With each passing year, we seem to pay more for less security. We have more people looking over our shoulders to see that we comply with rules that shift as rapidly as changing tides and that are as complicated as tax codes. We see the miracles of technology, knowing that those who can pay—not necessarily those who will benefit—will be their beneficiaries. We hope that the insurance lottery has given us a policy that will cover this service.

Policy experts tend to blame our reliance on private, fee-for-service medicine. But all Western countries, regardless of their delivery systems, are facing similar problems of rising demand and costs. A 1993 joint study by Andersen Consulting and Burson-Marsteller that surveyed nearly 3,000 health-care professionals, purchasers, suppliers, manufacturers, and policy experts in ten countries found that each country is facing similar challenges. The recession that hit most Western countries aggravated cost pressures by squeezing the general tax or employment-based revenues that support health systems worldwide.

Every system, including the ones that tend to be most admired, is running into problems. In Japan, nurses walked out to protest low wages and frequent night call. In 1992, French medical unions voted to strike following a law aimed at curbing health-care costs. The same year, the German parliament passed a legislative package intended to cut nearly $7 billion a year in health-care costs that included fee cuts for doctors, hospitals, and pharmacists as well as higher out-of-pocket costs for patients. And nearly one third of Canadian doctors have referred patients out of the country for treatment, according to a survey of doctors in the United States, western Germany, and Canada.

Even though foreign health-care systems are running into problems for many of the same reasons that we are—like expensive technology and aging populations—it's still worth looking at their systems. Comparison with other countries can give us insight into the particular American rendition of medicine—and our possible solutions.

A look at hospital statistics offers a glimpse at how facile answers are unlikely to be successful. It's tempting to think that slashing hospital admissions would yield significant cost savings, since 40 percent of our health-care budget goes to hospital costs. But a comparison with seven other Western countries on the availability and use of hospital beds shows that despite the highest per capita health-care spending in the world, we already rank low in many hospital parameters. Only Canada has relatively fewer beds per 1,000 population. Our admission rate is relatively low. And our average length of stay is the lowest of all the countries—just over nine days in 1990. By contrast, Japan's average length of hospital stay topped fifty days, even though health care accounts for only 8 percent of Japan's gross national product. Where we are highest, however, is the number of employees per bed.

Although the comparison looks only at certain hospital statistics, it's probably safe to infer several points. Our system is administratively top-heavy and technologically intensive, making it reliant on a large labor force. One recent study found that administrative costs accounted for one out of every four dollars spent in U.S. hospitals, and that over a twenty-year period, in which hospital admissions had fallen by roughly half, the number of hospital employees had nearly tripled. Another study comparing hospital expenses in the United States and Canada found that U.S. costs for each admission were much higher, despite shorter hospital stays. In addition to high administrative costs, the study cited excess capacity in medical technology. Ironically, the push to shorten hospital stays means that we have required many services to be available on short notice, services that demand hiring more staff. And the high-capacity use of technology in Canada may involve a trade-off of patients waiting longer but having more experienced personnel perform the tests. Although all industrialized countries have the same technology available—sometimes it is even introduced earlier abroad because of more relaxed malpractice climates—we use it more often. California alone has at least 400 MRI machines for a population of 31 million, while all of Canada has only 20 for its 27 million citizens. We have half the world's CAT scanners.

Greater health-care satisfaction abroad is probably due to a higher sense of security. Foreign governments tend to lend a protective hand, even when the system is basically private, as it is in France, Germany, and Holland. Although people may complain about amenities, like un-air-conditioned hospital rooms or crowded clinics, they feel that they won't fall through the safety net.

Many countries even offer a wider range of services despite lower total costs. People abroad don't worry about arbitrary benefits or going bankrupt. In Austria, vasectomies and vasectomy reversals and in vitro fertilization were covered at a time when most U.S. insurance plans wouldn't pay for these services.

In England, homeopathic medicine is provided as well as traditional medicine under the National Health Service. In England and Holland, there were tracking systems to ensure that children were immunized. France, Japan, England, and Holland provided home visits for newborns. Germany paid for cures taken at spas, for the healing power of mud baths. People in stressful occupations were entitled to four weeks at a sanitarium if their physician deemed it preventive care. Others could visit a spa every three years for a couple of weeks. Germans also visited their doctors more often than Americans—eleven times a year on average, which was double our rate, according to this study.

Foreign governments have tried to place a universal medical safety net under their citizens. Until our recent debate, we have not considered universal protection since Harry Truman was president nearly fifty years ago.

The systems vary from country to country. Without getting bogged down in the details of all, it's worth looking at some. Many countries, including Japan, France, and Germany, mix public and private elements. French physicians tend to be private solo practitioners, working with a fee-for-service system. Patients pay the full fee directly, and they are then reimbursed by insurance (generally a combination of social security insurance and supplemental health insurance). Only one percent of the population is estimated to be uninsured. Funding is primarily through payroll taxes, with a total of 16 percent of wages going to supporting health care. The majority of physicians, those who are *conventionnés,* accept a government-regulated, uniform fee schedule—roughly twenty dollars for a generalist's office visit and twenty-eight dollars for a specialist's. It is not "first-franc" coverage, except with serious conditions. While patients pay 30 percent of routine office visits, they pay nothing for serious illnesses like cancer and AIDS, or for services like maternity care. The government sets global budgets for most hospitals and negotiates drug prices with the manufacturers. Although the French system is a hodgepodge of private and government initiatives, the government has guaranteed an accessible, predictable system.

Germany, too, mixes public and private. More than 1,200 nonprofit sickness funds channel revenues collected from employers and employees to eighteen regional associations of ambulatory-care doctors. In 1989, the combined tax on wages averaged nearly 13 percent. Germans earning above a certain income could choose between staying in their sickness fund or buying private insurance, but roughly 90 percent of the population chose to stay in the public domain—undoubtedly because re-entry into the public plan is difficult for those who leave. Unemployed and retired Germans remain members of sickness funds, although their premiums are subsidized by other sources. The doctors' associations set fee schedules, including reimbursement rates for hospitals. The German system offers universal access to a comprehensive set of benefits that includes burial allowances, maternity benefits, and paid leave for parents needing time off work to take care of a sick child.

Other countries are basically government-run, single-payer systems. But within this framework, there are many variations. Funding sources vary. Some, like Australia, use a designated income tax. Others, like New Zealand, draw from general tax revenues. Payment systems vary. Canada relies on fee-for-service payment to doctors; Britain uses capitation fees that are paid to general practitioners. The degree of centralization also varies. Canada uses decentralized partnerships between the provinces and the federal government. Britain uses a centralized National Health Service.

Despite these variations, common threads emerge that differentiate foreign systems from ours. Virtually every country uses generalists as the bedrock of health care. In other countries, however, they maintain a degree of clinical autonomy that's vanishing here. They also enjoy a higher level of prestige and have a clearer identity. In Canada, general medicine is ruled by the College of Family Physicians, whereas in the United States primary care is scattered under the banners of several professional societies, like the American College of Physicians, the American Society of Internal Medicine, the American Academy of Family Physicians, the American Academy of Pediatrics, and the American College of Obstetrics and Gynecology. Adding to the confusion, internists in the United States function both as generalists and specialists, whereas in Canada they are clearly differentiated as specialists, leaving Canadian generalists their distinct turf. The pay gap between Canadian generalists and specialists is roughly 30 percent, whereas in the United States it can easily be 200 percent.

In many countries, hospital physicians are salaried, with little or no crossover into the realm of outpatient medicine. This is basically true for Britain, France, and Germany. The drawback for patients is that they are no longer treated by someone with whom they have a long-standing relationship. And they probably have no choice in their hospital doctor. But in many ways, particularly in cities where there are lots of doctors, it is a more efficient system. Doctors no longer have to be in two places at once. And hospital doctors, who may do costly procedures like angioplasties, then have no fee-for-service incentive to do so, since they are salaried. For patients, it's a trade-off. They might be guaranteed a higher level of hospital medicine, but they may also find it frightening to have their care managed entirely by strangers.

Doctors abroad often have an institutionalized role in the creation of health policy. In this country, they are increasingly excluded. Even Cuba, a country with limited resources, understood the importance of meshing clinical experience and policy decisions. In the early 1980s, Cuban hospital administrators were physicians who had additional training as administrators. In Britain, the National Health Service began an experiment that allowed some general practices to negotiate with hospitals and laboratories. Doctors gained control over how services were allocated. In Germany, regional medical associations are part of the country's legal structure. In Japan, the Japanese Medical Association has two seats in parliament. At a 1990 conference comparing health care in Britain, Canada, and the United States, both the Canadians and the Britons said that physicians in their countries wouldn't tolerate the micromanagement foisted on the medical profession by third parties in this country. The involvement of physicians in setting medical policy, in determining what services are worth paying for, may explain why benefits abroad are less arbitrary. Here we have relied on insurance companies run by businessmen to tell us what is worth financing.

Medical education in many other countries, including Germany, France, and Canada, is either free or provided with minimal tuition costs. Unlike in the United States, where medical students must look first to repaying their personal debt, new medical graduates abroad can more readily concentrate on their obligations to society. The give-and-take is institutionalized in other ways as well. Under Britain's National Health Service, general practitioners who are not salaried but receive a set capitation fee for each patient in the practice are entitled to six weeks of paid vacation annually, paid sabbaticals, and a pension from the NHS on retirement. Here doctors are left to fend for themselves.

But it isn't just the emphasis on technology and the more chaotic delivery system that differentiate U.S. medical care from that in foreign countries. Malpractice litigation looms here with a presence unheard of abroad. Despite that, our health statistics are worse than in many foreign countries.

In the United States, we take it as given that health-care businesses must be able to reap jackpot rewards, that innovation is sparked by a wildcatting instinct. Yet other countries with government-run health care have pioneered many developments. Britain, where the first test-tube baby was born, is developing robots for surgery. Surgeons in Canada are using robots to treat complicated neurological tumors. Yet both countries have nationalized health-care systems. Britain also spends relatively little on drugs yet maintains a high research budget for pharmaceuticals.

Although we should look abroad for ideas and better understanding of our strengths and weaknesses, we need to understand that they can't be simply transposed. Each country has evolved a medical system in keeping with its specific society.

Japan's health-care system is based on the concept of *wa*—the harmony of the group. Prevention and community health contribute to Japan's having the lowest infant mortality rate and longest life expectancy in the industrialized world. Theirs is a paternalistic system, and one where patients wait hours for appointments that last only a few minutes. Physicians are generally unquestioned—either by patients or by research looking for outcomes, largely because of the Confucian principle of *jin*, or paternalistic love. The "doctors' margin," a markup on drugs prescribed and dispensed by physicians, accounts for a significant percentage of doctors' incomes in Japan but would be considered unethical here. And, in fact, it does lead to overmedication. Organ transplantation is virtually nonexistent in Japan, partly because of Buddhist beliefs that the soul cannot go to heaven (and therefore toward reincarnation) until the heart stops beating, making it difficult to get organs from someone who is brain dead, but whose heart is still beating. Death is something to hide, therefore it's unlikely— even in the absence of social unity—that patients would band together to lobby for spending on specific diseases. It is a system that has little bearing on ours, except to cause envy—for the near-universal access, long lifespans, and all at a cost of only 8 percent of Japan's GNP.

Professional traditions influence subtle aspects of health care, like what drugs are popular. Medical prescribing habits show cultural variations. German physicians like combination medications, whereas British doctors regard them as unscientific and even unsafe. The French are the world's greatest consumers of Valium-like drugs, with one in three persons taking a tranquilizer or similar drug. Yet across the Channel, only one in ten people take such drugs.

Each country must respond to its specific health needs. Because of immigration, the rates of tuberculosis are climbing by as much as 33 percent annually across Europe. We in the United States have an epidemic of violence-related illnesses because guns are widely available. Yet each country also faces the chronic illnesses that are common to aging, affluent societies. Each must find solutions in keeping with national traditions, both within and without the health-care system.

Holistic Healing—A Metaphor for Problem Solving

Reforming Americans' health care will require a dose of New Age medicine—holistic healing. Medical practice is like an ecosystem, in which all parts are interdependent and dynamic. Instead of targeting the components of health care piecemeal, we need to nudge all players toward reform, toward the ultimate goals of stabilizing costs, providing care for everyone, ensuring medical advances, and taking the anxiety out of the system.

An experiment carried out in Maine offers a preview of such "interdisciplinary" reform. The state's legislature limited malpractice liability for doctors who followed clinical guidelines. In a five-year experiment involving obstetrician-gynecologists, radiologists, emergency medicine doctors, and anesthesiologists, doctors who followed the guidelines could have malpractice suits dismissed before trial. Although any recommendation to dismiss the claim would be nonbinding—patients could still choose to initiate a trial—pretrial findings would be admissible in court. The policy was aimed at slashing the costs of defensive medicine, estimated to run between $4 billion and $25 billion a year. The main reason cited by doctors for incurring these costs was their uncertainty about the standard of care to which they would be held in the event of a suit.

The plan involved the cooperation of the medical and business communities, along with the recognition that practicing doctors should have strong input. Intended to take effect if 50 percent of each specialty agreed, the plan actually enlisted the support of 80 percent of doctors in the four specialties. Guidelines were set by local doctors, not imposed by policy experts or academic physicians. The five-year demonstration project covering twenty procedures in the four specialties started January 1, 1992. Although Maine is smaller than most states and more homogeneous than many, this offers a model for the process of reform. If the guidelines work, they could have a domino effect: lowering malpractice insurance costs, lowering medical costs, lowering patients' insurance costs, and increasing the ranks of the insured.

Other plans have also shown encouraging results. Harvard's chiefs of anesthesia developed practice guidelines to improve patient care and lower malpractice rates. Comparing the periods before and after the guidelines were implemented showed dramatic results. From 1976 to 1985, the average anesthesia-related claim was $153,000. In the three years after guidelines went into effect, the average cost of each claim was $34,000. Not only did patient care improve, but Harvard anesthesiologists saw their 1989 insurance rates drop by nearly one third from those of the previous year. Whether reform initiatives are broad-based or limited to one network of hospitals, we need to be able to tackle several angles of health-care reform at once.

Several aspects of the medical profession need to be revamped, including the skewed ratio of generalists and specialists, the great income divide between the two, and perhaps even the question of who should be our generalists.

If we are to revive the generalist, we have to recast him as someone whose broad range of knowledge can cope with most medical ailments rather than as someone who lacks the expertise to perform high-tech miracles. Policy experts have proposed several ways of drawing medical students into primary-care tracks, like forgiving tuition costs and limiting access to specialist training programs. But they overlook an inexpensive tool: the enthusiastic mentor. The reality today, however, is that medical students are staring into the eyes of disenchanted mid-career role models. The forty-something generation of doctors remembers being trained by role models who loved their work. But the forty-something generation of generalists now sees mountains of paperwork, a hostile practice environment, growing social ills that have been left to become chronic medical problems, and a growing disparity of income with their procedurally oriented colleagues. Incentives won't work without fixing the drawbacks of practice.

One of those drawbacks is the great income divide between procedure-oriented specialists and non-procedure-oriented generalists. The Harvard economist who designed the revamped Medicare payments to physicians that was intended partly to redress this wrong, warned that the current system "produces unreasonably low levels of payment overall, which could dissuade those considering a career in medicine from entering the field." Primary-care doctors have often earned less than the pharmaceutical representatives who pitch drugs to them. In the early 1990s, the 50,000 salespeople for the pharmaceutical industry were estimated to earn between $60,000 and $150,000 each. It would be hard to argue that a "drug detail" person or his supervisor should earn more than a pediatrician or internist. Although the insurance industry underwrote the financial schism within medicine, the profession itself will have to grapple with what differential is fair. And the public has to realize that cutting doctors' incomes by 20 percent would lower health-care costs by less than 2 percent. It would not solve the cost problem.

Another question that we need to raise, beyond the generalist-specialist ratio, is who should deliver primary care? Some people feel that workers with lesser training, like nurse practitioners, could do the same work at lower cost. While they certainly could provide services like immunizations, I think it would be a mistake not to have primary-care physicians as the backbone of health care, as they are in every other country. I think we should consider using more family practitioners rather than internists, pediatricians, and gynecologists to provide first-line coverage. Particularly in underserved areas, their broad range of skills could serve the population well. Pediatricians, internists, and gynecologists could shift away from routine care to specialty care, for which they are trained. Well-child care, family planning, routine GYN exams, and care of common maladies like hypertension could be done by family practitioners. The sharper boundary between generalist and specialist might lead to a split between outpatient and in-hospital medicine (except in rural areas with physician shortages), much as it does in other countries. Hospitalized patients might lose continuity of care, but they might also benefit from greater expertise. There are clearly compromises to be made.

Doctors also need more coordinated, ongoing medical education that is both outcome- and cost-oriented. For instance, the recent rise in tuberculosis cases which has paralleled the rise in AIDS and homelessness warrants updates for physicians in affected areas. But a study by the major TB-referral hospital suggested that community doctors were failing to offer good first-line treatment. A study of thirty-five patients with multi-drug-resistant TB admitted to the National Jewish Center for Immunology and Respiratory Medicine in Denver found that twenty-eight patients had been mismanaged. The cost of treatment, which might otherwise have been relatively cheap, came to $180,000 per patient.

Practice research needs to be tailored to the realities of delivering care, not some standard that is impractical. There needs to be a more active feedback loop between practicing doctors and the academic medical community. For instance, the TB study—done in an academic setting—could be used to suggest that it is cost-effective to have pulmonary specialists rather than general physicians treat TB in urban areas with high rates of drug-resistant TB. A feedback loop between academics and local doctors could promote more efficient use of academic centers as backup, particularly if hospital-based experts could be used as curbside consultants to provide informal second opinions. For instance, fax machines can be used to have a cardiologist take a look at a cardiogram for the generalist who is unsure of its interpretation.

The medical profession also needs more outcomes research—which looks at the effectiveness of treatment—to help guide its decisions. It needs to look at procedures that cost a lot and that are done frequently, and it needs to look at the issue of marginal benefits—those situations with such a low chance of success that treatment isn't justified. While academic medicine can do the studies looking at marginal benefits, our society needs to face the issue. When is something too costly, when does it have such a low margin of success that it simply isn't worth it? The question has undertones of rationing, but it is a principle that pervades our lives—although we feel that medical decisions should be spared such relativism. Anyone thinking of moving into a bigger house would weigh the pros and cons, perhaps deciding that it's not worth it because he can't afford something sufficiently bigger or it would mean moving out of our familiar neighborhood. We make trade-offs in all aspects of our lives, but pretend that such trade-offs don't exist in health care. They do.

Doctors can supply the medical data, but this is a debate for the public. We will simply go bankrupt if we aim to provide all services to all people regardless of cost or likelihood of success, no matter how much or little we pay doctors. Our ability to diagnose illness has outstripped our ability to treat in many cases. Do we always need to know? A certain treatment may only add three months of life but cost $20,000. Do we really want to do this? These are decisions that the public needs to consider—not just doctors, politicians, and health insurers—since it is ultimately up to the people to decide how much money they want to spend.

If the concept of marginal benefits is to be addressed, lawyers also will have to be involved. Without a change in the legal system—which defends every individual's right to maximum treatment—it is unlikely that we will make rational use of this concept. That would be unfortunate, because it is an area in which there is room to maneuver. If the idea is attacked as the first step on the "slippery slope to rationing," we might do better to see it as the first step in guaranteeing access to all.

Whether doctors are more symptom or cause of the current crisis, it is true that physicians failed to take the lead in reform at a time when as insiders they knew that there were significant problems. For some doctors, it may have been greed, or at least the coincidence of private gain and public policy. For others, it was simply burying their heads in the sand. They didn't have the time, energy, or inclination to broaden their horizons past their individual practices. Then one day they were jogged into alertness by a disgruntled public, an activist insurance industry, and unsympathetic legislators.

In addition to changing the way doctors train, practice, and are paid, we also have to change their working environment. Partly that means changing the legal climate. In the Maine experiment, malpractice insurers worried they might be held liable retroactively for claims in which guidelines were the defense, if a defense based on these guidelines was subsequently found to be unconstitutional. That is a strong disincentive for using guidelines. The threat of malpractice hangs like a punitive cloud over the heads of practicing doctors, acting as a strong disincentive for doctors to moderate their use of diagnostic technology. Why try to control costs by putting oneself at risk? Malpractice litigation reinforces the maximal and indiscriminate use of expensive technology.

In the brave new world of "managed care," the issue of malpractice is becoming more complicated. Doctors often bear full responsibility, even though their decisions are shaped by an HMO's directives. In response to this, some people have suggested "enterprise liability," which shifts the burden from the doctor to the institution or insurers. Perhaps tempting at first glance, this is a potential land mine. A doctor who accepts complicated cases might become a liability to the HMO. Malpractice suits might become the reason to unload him—and his costly patients. We will have to resolve these legal issues if we are to move forward with health-care reform.

Our legislators will also have to take greater responsibility for standing up to their electorate if science doesn't back what is politically expedient. Seeking to reform health care, they will have to shy away from simplistic arguments and keep their eyes open for unforeseen consequences of change. An example, unrelated to the medical world, of how good intentions go awry, is a government policy of giving businesses tax credits for hiring the poor. Although nobody would question the noble intention of the goal, reality turned out to be a different story. The tax incentive was called among the "most wasteful of all programs" because the companies, notably profitable national fast-food chains, would have hired the same workers anyway—but without a $2,400 tax break for each "targeted" worker.

Trying to cut costs, legislators can enact some measures that don't involve structural reform. Sin taxes are a recurrent idea. For every 10 percent price hike on cigarettes, the National Cancer Institute estimated that adult consumption drops 4 percent. As of 1992, we had the second-lowest cigarette tax among nineteen countries. Denmark topped the list with a tax of more than four dollars a pack—ours was fifty-one cents. Not only do sin taxes generate revenue, but they discourage harmful and costly habits (although some people point out that nonsmokers live longer, ultimately costing more money than smokers who die young).

But sin taxes won't raise or save enough money to avoid altering our delivery system. We have two basic choices about moving from where we are to where we want to be. One would be incremental changes, closing loopholes. We could start by eliminating the tax-deductibility of health insurance (rather than extending it to all), standardizing benefit packages, requiring individuals to buy insurance or join an HMO, and bringing ERISA health benefits under the control of state insurance departments. There are a host of changes that could stabilize our current plight. Or we could try a more cataclysmic overhaul. Regardless of what we do, we need to reduce our indiscriminate appetite for more health care and more high technology. And we need to move resources out of sinkholes and into areas where they will make a difference.

Whatever way we go, we must design something for the long haul, something that is theoretically stable and adaptable to the changing realities of care. A report on Germany's efforts to reform its health care found that "one of the most important lessons from the German experience is that health-care reform is a continuous process. As the United States moves toward comprehensive health-care reform, it should incorporate enough flexibility in its system to ensure responsiveness to a constantly changing health market."

Epilogue

As THIS BOOK GOES TO PRESS, the Clinton health plan is on the table. While few people would deny that we have to do something, many disagree about what we should do—whether we have a crisis or a system that merely needs improvement.

The Clintons deserve credit for making health-care reform a national priority and for recognizing that it must be dealt with on a federal level, rather than left to the fragmentary efforts of states.

But there are many disturbing features of the Clinton plan, beginning with the task force's veil of secrecy that masked any real discussion of underlying issues before legislation was drafted. Whatever public meetings took place looked more like staged publicity events than genuine debates about the substance of health-care reform. While the task force justified its need for concealment by claiming that seclusion gave the reformers room to maneuver without pressure from special interest groups, the secrecy also masked their weaknesses. This was not a group with long-standing involvement in the delivery of health care. At the helm were businessmen, lawyers, policy analysts, and politicians. The team avoided public scrutiny before completing its crash-course in health care.

The 1,342-page Health Security Act that emerged from the task force does address the key issue of universal coverage, but it does so by creating a new and immensely complicated bureaucracy. The proposed legislation creates regional health alliances at the local level and establishes the National Health Board at the federal level. Trusting that such a politically appointed bureaucracy would be efficient—either economically or medically—requires a giant leap of faith.

Regional alliances, the linchpins of the Clinton proposal, are a potential nightmare of bureaucratic and political wrangling. Although intended mainly as a way of buying insurance and evaluating different health plans—like a giant corporate benefits office—the alliances are unlikely to work well. For a start, the rules that define them are overwhelmingly complex, as the following excerpt suggests: "Plan Sponsor of a Multiemployer

205

Plan—A plan sponsor described in section 3(16)(B)(iii) of Employee Retirement Security Act of 1974, but only with respect to a group health plan that is a multiemployer plan (as defined in subsection (e)(4)) maintained by the sponsor and only if—" That's only one paragraph from 106 pages that describe the form and function of the alliances.

But the problem isn't purely technical. Underlying the alliances is a belief in "managed competition," private plans vying for customers under government supervision. These plans provide total health care for a set fee, linking insurer and providers into a single unit.

Enthusiasts of managed competition cite the success of Cal-PERS—the California Public Employees' Retirement Systems that pools public employees in California for buying health insurance. But they may be overstating the benefits, according to the Government Accounting Office. While it's true that 1993 CalPERS premiums increased by only 1.4 percent, and 1992 premiums by 6.1 percent, it was a very different story from 1989 through 1991. During those years, premiums jumped by 16.7 percent annually—which was higher than the national average. The GAO warned, in a recent report, that "it is inappropriate to characterize CalPERS' recent experience as an indicator of the potential effectiveness of managed competition in constraining health insurance premiums."

At the federal level, the Clinton plan creates a National Health Board of seven members to be appointed by the president, with the advice and consent of the Senate. Unless board members have both the knowledge and independence of someone like former surgeon general Dr. C. Everett Koop, we are all at risk. History suggests that his combination of expertise, objectivity, and willingness to do battle may be rare. Regional alliances and the National Health Board are likely to politicize health care—a problem that we certainly don't need.

The plan has plenty of other structural problems. It leaves the current segmentation of the insurance market intact, setting the stage for continued cost-shifting and high administrative overhead. Self-insured companies, Medicare, Medicaid, the Veterans' Health Service, and the Indian Health Service will still exist. But as two communities—the city of Rochester, New York, and the state of Hawaii—show, unification of the insurance market is critical to providing universal access and cost control.

Although the Clinton plan offers universal access, this applies only to legal residents. But some states, like California, Texas, and New York, have many illegal immigrants who may account for a disproportionate share of some public health problems, like tuberculosis. Their exclusion raises humanitarian and practical concerns. Many are children—do we really want to turn them down? If immigrants carry infections like TB, don't we want to minimize the spread of disease?

The plan maintains the employment-health insurance link. Since employers would generally pick up 80 percent of the health insurance tab, Americans will remain oblivious to the costs of health care. That's a big mistake. Not only do workers actually pay through lower wages, but deluded by the impression that health care is free, they have no incentive to lower the demand for services. Unless we begin to reduce demand, we will one day ration health care by inconvenience.

The Health Security Act maintains the basic financial inequities of our current system—probably to avoid the political nemesis of taxes. Except for the poor and the "recapture of certain health subsidies received by high-income individuals," the plan has no real tie-in to personal income. The CEO earning $2 million pays essentially the same for his health insurance as the janitor earning $20,000—assuming they choose the same plan.

Apart from the structural problems, there are medical ones as well. Although the plan rightly includes preventive services, there is a nagging sense that the plan's architects are trying to persuade us that these services will help cut our health-care budget. Providing these basic services is part of rational and humane medical care, but it is unlikely to reduce our reliance on high-tech medicine. The difficult question for our health-care future isn't "How do we improve the delivery of preventive services?" but "How do we learn to use expensive, high-tech medicine selectively?" The plan avoids the question that is at the root of our health-care problems. Neither the AMA's approach of decrying limits on health expenditures nor politicians' claims that costs can be limited without restricting services is true. We need to admit that there is a middle ground, even if it is thorny. This is the time for that debate.

The Health Security Act doesn't invite participation from doctors in policy or payment decisions. In fact, health-care providers are explicitly excluded from the boards of directors that run the regional alliances, because the plan labels this a conflict of interest. Excluding those with the greatest expertise from making decisions is absurd—it's like ruling out lawyers as lawmakers or soldiers as military strategists. When a White House spokesman defended this position by saying that the alliances were purely insurance-purchasing cooperatives, he confirmed a huge problem in health care today—keeping the providers out of the policy loop. Unless we coordinate clinical and financial decisions, we cannot make rational decisions about what health care can and should offer.

Many view this plan as a boon for managed care, specifically for the insurance companies that will run these plans. What happened to the analyses by the Congressional Budget Office and the General Accounting Office? These analyses suggested the biggest savings would be achieved by HMOs *with* walls, which may be more restrictive than what most Americans want. These reports questioned long-term savings from managed care.

We haven't even begun to address questions of cost. Since cost is ultimately the root of the access problem for most Americans, failure to come up with realistic numbers could be a disaster. At some point financial reality is bound to intrude—even if it doesn't at the time legislation is passed. There isn't enough waste and fraud in the system to make cutting costs painless—an assumption that underlies managed competition. This plan has a politician's stamp of promises without compromise. We get universal coverage—that's an extra 39 million people. We also get increased services for those who are already insured. Medicare recipients, who now aren't covered for outpatient drugs, would be. Younger Americans are promised routine physicals—a popular idea for which there is little medical value. And the deficit is reduced.

While the Clintons have dismissed a single-payer system as politically not feasible, we should at least discuss the benefits. It has two assets which are among the most desirable of any system. Single-payer offers the greatest patient flexibility and the lowest plan overhead. These are features that should at least be considered.

A cataclysmic overhaul that fails may leave us worse off than we are. We could wind up spending more for less. We could lose the technical innovation and the rapid access that most Americans have enjoyed. These pitfalls are not a justification to let things remain as they are. They are merely the reasons to have an honest discussion in an open forum. We need to understand the problems before we impose the solution.

Notes

Introduction: Medicine Has Changed

xii Anders, George, "McDonald's Methods Come to Medicine As Chains Acquire Physicians' Practices." Wall Street Journal, August 24, 1993:B1.

xiii BlueCross BlueShield Association, Environmental Analysis, 1992: 4.

xiii Robert Pear, "Health-Care Costs Up Sharply Again, Posing New Threat," New York Times, January 5, 1993: A1.

xiii Simon Francis, "U.S. Industrial Outlook 1993—Health and Medical Services." U.S. Department of Commerce, 42–44.

xiii "Health Care, the Job Builder," New York Times, June 6, 1993: F13.

xiii The Learning Annex. January/February 1993: 3.

xiii Commerce Department fax, January 25, 1994.

xiii "HCA Chairman Got Compensation in 1992 Totaling $127 Million," Wall Street Journal, March 24, 1993: B5.

xiii "Sign of the Times," American Medical News, May 18, 1992: 24.

xiv Insider Trading Spotlight, Wall Street Journal, May 13, 1992: C23; June 24, 1992: C19; June 10, 1992: C25; June 17, 1992: C21; August 19, 1992: C19; October 21, 1992: C17.

xiv "Government Finds Wider Gap on Financing of Pensions," New York Times, November 23, 1993: D12.

xv Jeff Gerth, "U.S. Pension Agency Is in Deep Trouble, Economists Warn," New York Times, December 20, 1992: A1.

xv Paul Krugman, "Like It or Not, the Income Gap Yawns," Wall Street Journal, May 21, 1992: A13.

xv Children's Defense Fund, personal communication, October 1993.

xv Celia Dugger, "Their Wages Low, Single Mothers Get Little Help," New York Times, March 31, 1992: A1.

xv "Record 25 Million People on Food Stamp Rolls," New York Times, March 29, 1992: A17.

xv Jacques Steinberg, "U.S. Social Well-Being Is Rated Lowest Since Study Began in 1970," New York Times, October 5, 1992: B6.

xv Robert Gellman, "Prescribing Privacy: The Uncertain Role of the Physician in the Protection of Patient Privacy," North Carolina Law Review 62 (1984): 267.

Chapter 1: Costs—Headed Higher

5 Jeffrey Groeger et al., "Descriptive Analysis of Critical Care Units in the United States." Critical Care Medicine 21 (1993): 279–91.

5 Congressional Health Care Workshops, September, 1993, chart 5.

5 Health Care Financing Administration, Health Care Financing Review, HCFA Publication No. 03335, U.S. Government Printing Office (Winter 1992): 162.

5 U.S. Industrial Outlook 1994, U.S. Commerce Department: 42–1.

5 Michael De Courcy Hinds, "Study Sees Pain Ahead in States' Budgets," New York Times, July 27, 1993: A8.

5 Eli Ginzberg, "Health Care Reform—Where Are We and Where Should We Be Going?" *New England Journal of Medicine* 327 (1992): 1310–12.

5 U.S. General Accounting Office, "Health Care Reform," December 1992: 6.

6 *Health Care Financing Review,* 1992: 163.

6 Eli Ginzberg, "Physician Supply Policies and Health Reform," *JAMA* 268 (1992): 3115–18.

7 Medicare: Excessive Payments Support the Proliferation of Costly Technology." GAO Report, GAO/HRD-92-59, May 1992: 3.

7 R. Berenson and J. Holahan, "Sources of Growth in Medicare Physician Expenditures," *JAMA* 267 (1992): 687–91.

7 "Mammograms on Rise," *New York Times,* April 29, 1992: C13.

8 Stephen Moore, "European State-Funded Health Systems Come Under Fire for Skyrocketing Costs," *Wall Street Journal,* May 4, 1993: A14.

8 Robert Pear, "States Are Moving to Re-regulation on Health Costs," *New York Times,* May 11, 1992: A1.

8 "Economic Implications of Rising Health Care Costs," Congressional Budget Office, October 1992: 22, 25–26.

8 Joseph Newhouse, "Iconoclastic View," *Health Affairs,* Supplement, 1993: 160–61.

9 Jeanne Kassler, "New Weapon Cleans Coronary Arteries," *New York Times,* July 14, 1991: LI 8.

10 Ashby Jordan, "Hospital Charges for Laparoscopic and Open Cholecystectomy" (letter), *JAMA* 266 (1991): 3425.

10 Antonio Legorreta et al., "Increased Cholecystectomy Rate After the Introduction of Laparoscopic Cholecystectomy," *JAMA* 270 (1993): 1429–32.

11 BlueCross BlueShield Association, Environmental Analysis, 1992: 31.

11 Congressional Budget Office, "Economic Implications of Rising Health Care Costs," October 1992: 4.

12 BlueCross BlueShield Association, Environmental Analysis, 1992: 19.

12 Thomas Burton, "Firms That Promise Lower Medical Bills May Increase Them," *Wall Street Journal,* July 28, 1992: A1.

12 Steffie Woolhandler and David Himmelstein, "The Deteriorating Administrative Efficiency of the U.S. Health Care System," *New England Journal of Medicine,* 324 (1991): 1253–58.

12 Special Committee on Aging, U.S. Senate, "The Drug Manufacturing Industry: A Prescription for Profits," U.S. Government Printing Office, Washington, 1991.

14 Congressional Budget Office, "Economic Implications of Rising Health Care Costs," October, 1992: 41.

14 Health and Human Services news releases, February 19, 1993, and March 17, 1993.

14 Peter Magowan, "A Great Prognosis for 'Play or Pay,'" *Wall Street Journal,* March 26, 1992: A15.

15 Doron Levin, "G.M. Orders Staff to Pay Part of Health-Care Cost," *New York Times,* August 26, 1992: D3.

15 Bill Clinton, "The Clinton Health Care Plan," *New England Journal of Medicine* 327 (1992): 804–7.

15 Congressional Budget Office, "Economic Implications of Rising Health Care Costs," October 1992: 5, 47.

15 Elaine Povich, "The Medical-Care Cost Squeeze," *Chicago Tribune,* May 27, 1991: 1.

15 Thomas Bodenheimer, "Underinsurance in America," *New England Journal of Medicine* 327 (1992): 274–77.

15 The Henry J. Kaiser Foundation and The Commonwealth Fund, "Americans' Health Care Concerns: A National Survey," April 8, 1992.

15 John Iglehart, "The American Health Care System: Community Hospitals," *New England Journal of Medicine* 329 (1993): 372–76.

15 Joseph Sullivan, "Judge Stays Rate Ruling for Hospitals," *New York Times,* June 5, 1992: B1.

16 David Eddy, "Three Battles to Watch in the 1990s," *JAMA* 270 (1993): 520–26.

Chapter 2: Access—More and More Are Losing It

18 Micki Siegel, "Helping My Friend Sent Us Both to Jail," *Good Housekeeping,* May 1993: 153–59.

18 "Health Insurance: Vulnerable Payers Lose Billions to Fraud and Abuse," General Accounting Office, GAO/HRD-92-69, May, 1992: 20.

18 Tamar Lewin, "Health-Care System Is Issue in Jailing of Uninsured Patient," *New York Times,* January 8, 1993: A10.

19 Victor Fuchs, "Dear President Clinton," *JAMA* 269 (1993): 1678–79.

19 *Employment and Health Benefits,* Institute of Medicine (Washington, D.C., National Academy Press: 1993), 109.

19 Jennifer Dixon, "U.S. Health Care. 1: The Access Problem," *BMJ* 305 (1992): 817–19.

19 Congressional Budget Office, "Economic Implications of Rising Health Care Costs," October 1992: 6.

19 Thomas Bodenheimer, "Underinsurance in America," *New England Journal of Medicine* 327 (1992): 274–77.

20 Sara Rosenbaum et al., "Children and Health Insurance," Children's Defense Fund, January 1992.

20 Robert Pear, "Fewer Are Insured for Medical Care," *New York Times,* December 15, 1993: A24.

20 Thomas Bodenheimer, "Underinsurance in America," *New England Journal of Medicine* 327 (1992): 274–77.

20 P. A. Singer and F. H. Lowy, "Rationing, Patient Preferences and Cost of Care at the End of Life," *Archives of Internal Medicine* 152 (1992): 478–80.

21 Nicola Clark, "The High Costs of Dying," *Wall Street Journal,* February 26, 1992: A12.

21 P. A. Singer and F. H. Lowy, "Rationing, Patient Preferences and Cost of Care at the End of Life," *Archives of Internal Medicine* 152 (1992): 478–80.

21 Claudia Moraine, "Save the Children," *American Medical News,* December 21, 1992: 24.

21 Sara Rosenbaum et al., "Children and Health Insurance," Children's Defense Fund, January 1992.

21 Gina Kolata, "Baby's Painful Two Years of Life Highlight the High Cost of Futile Care," *New York Times,* October 6, 1993: B7.

22 Joseph Tiang-Yau Liu and Sara Rosenbaum, "Medicaid and Childhood Immunizations: A National Study," Children's Defense Fund, January 1992.

22 Andrew Skolnick, "Should Insurance Cover Routine Immunizations?" *JAMA* 265 (1992): 2453–54.

23 Joseph Tiang-Yau Liu and Sara Rosenbaum, "Medicaid and Childhood Immunizations: A National Study," Children's Defense Fund, January 1992.

23 General Accounting Office. "Medicaid. HealthPASS: An Evaluation of a Managed Care Program for Certain Philadelphia Recipients," GAO/HRD-93-67, May 1993: 29–30.

24 Jeanne Kassler, "Managed Care—or Chaos?" *New York Magazine*, August 23, 1993: 44–50.

Chapter 3: Insurance—Now You See It, Now You Don't

25 Jeanne Kassler, "All About Health Insurance," *New York Magazine*, February 17, 1992: 48–51.

25 Milt Freudenheim, "The Unquiet Future of Commercial Health Insurance," *New York Times*, July 12, 1992: F11.

26 Personal communication, Bob Bennefield, Census Bureau, January 25, 1994.

26 Donald Light, "The Practice and Ethics of Risk-Related Health Insurance," *JAMA* 267 (1992): 2503–8.

26 Jennifer Dixon, "U.S. Health Care. 3: The Reform Problem," *BMJ*, 1992: 941–44.

27 Congressional Budget Office, "Economic Implications of Rising Health Care Costs," October 1992: 6.

27 John Goodman, "Health Insurance: States Can Help," *Wall Street Journal*, December 17, 1991: A20.

29 Ron Winslow, " 'House Calls' by Phone Seen Improving Care," *Wall Street Journal*, April 1, 1992: B1.

29 Elaine Power, "Home Drug Infusion Under Medicare," *JAMA* 279 (1993): 427.

29 Donald Light, "The Practice and Ethics of Risk-Related Health Insurance," *JAMA* 267 (1992): 2503–8.

29 "AIDS and Health Insurance: A Survey," Office of Technology Assessment, 1988.

29 Steffie Woolhandler and David Himmelstein, "The Deteriorating Administrative Efficiency of the U.S. Health Care System," *New England Journal of Medicine* 324 (1991): 1253–58.

29 "Report Details Spending of PA Blues Plans," *American Medical News*, August 3, 1992: 29.

30 Congressional Budget Office, "Economic Implications of Rising Health Care Costs," October 1992: 25.

30 John Ferguson et al., "Court-Ordered Reimbursement for Unproven Medical Technology," *JAMA* 269 (1993): 2116–21.

31 *The Bulletin*, New York State Insurance Department, April 1992.

31 Personal communication, 1992.

32 Robert Tomsho, "Consumers Squeezed as Insurers Dispute 'Usual and Customary' Medical Fees," *Wall Street Journal*, September 10, 1993: B1.

32 Jeanne Kassler, "All About Health Insurance," *New York Magazine*, February 17, 1992: 48–51.

32 "Hartford Life to Move $820 Million in Benefits," *New York Times*, September 15, 1993: D5.

33 Peter Kerr, "Insurers Faulted on Policy Switch," *New York Times*, April 22, 1992: A1.

33 National Association of Insurance Commissioners, news release, December 5, 1993.

33 Congressional Health Care Workshops, September 1993, chart 11.

34 Grace Monaco, director of legal and professional affairs, Candlelight Childhood Cancer Foundation, personal communication: September 30, 1993.

34 "Off-Label Drugs," General Accounting Office, GAO/PEMD-91-14, September, 1991: 3–4.

34 "Medical Testing and Health Insurance," U.S. Congress, Office of Technology Assessment, 1988: 3.

35 "Medical Testing and Health Insurance," U.S. Congress, Office of Technology Assessment, 1988: 8–12, 52–65.

35 Donald Light, "The Practice and Ethics of Risk-Related Health Insurance," *JAMA* 267 (1992): 2583–8.

35 Congressional Health Care Workshops, September, 1993, chart 17.

36 Mark Hall, "Reforming the Health Insurance Market," *New England Journal of Medicine* 326 (1992): 565–70.

36 Thomas Stoddard, "Now You're Insured, Now You're Not." *New York Times*, May 23, 1992: I23 (op-ed).

36 Edward Felsenthal, "Health Plans Are Self-Insured by More Firms," *Wall Street Journal*, November 11, 1992: B1.

37 Lawrence Gostin and Alan Widiss, "What's Wrong With the ERISA Vacuum?" *JAMA* 269 (1993): 2527–32.

37 Milt Freudenheim, "Employers Winning Right to Cut Back Medical Insurance," *New York Times*, March 29, 1992: A1.

37 Robert Pear, "Justices Leave Intact Ruling That Lets Business Cut Health Benefits," *New York Times*, November 10, 1992: A18.

38 Barry Meier, "Senate Panel Urges Action Against Phony Health Plans," *New York Times*, March 13, 1992: D1.

38 Peter Kerr, "3 Plead Guilty in Insurance Fraud Case," *New York Times*, December 30, 1992: D3.

38 Congressional Budget Office, "Economic Implications of Rising Health Care Costs," October 1992: 39.

38 Robert Ripstin, "Wrongheaded Hit at Retiree Benefits," *Wall Street Journal*, December 28, 1992: A10 (op-ed).

39 Uwe Reinhardt, "Financial Blows," *Health Affairs*, Supplement 1993: 183.

39 Scott McMurray, "DuPont to Cut Health Care Benefits in '94," *Wall Street Journal*, January 5, 1993: A3.

39 Mary Rowland, "Which Health Care Plan Will Pay?" *New York Times*, April 12, 1992: III 19.

40 Gerald Grumet, "Health Care Rationing Through Inconvenience," *New England Journal of Medicine* 321 (1992): 607–10.

40 Paul Dykewicz, "Group Wants Employers to Help Fund Health Care," *Journal of Commerce*, February 22, 1993: 7A.

Chapter 4: Losing the Family Doctor

42 William Carlos Williams, *The Doctor Stories* (New York: *New Directions*, 1984): xii.

43 Jack Colwill, "Where Have All the Primary Care Applicants Gone?" *New England Journal of Medicine* 326 (1992): 387–94.

43 Ronald Andersen et al., "National Study of Internal Medicine Manpower: XIX," *Annals of Internal Medicine* 117 (1992): 243–250.

43 Felicity Barringer, "Plastic Surgery: A Profession in Need of a Facelift?" *New York Times*, February 23, 1992: E5.

43 William Hsiao et al., "Assessing the Implementation of Physician-Payment Reform," *New England Journal of Medicine* 328 (1993): 928–33.

43 Howard Wolinsky, "Fed Up With Hassles and Financial Woes, Some General Internists Quit Their Practices," *ACP Observer* 12 (1992): 10.

44 Louis Harris and Associates, "Physicians and Medicare Fee Schedule: A Look at the Medicare Program and Other Payers in a Changing Practice Environment," February 1993: 8.

44 Barbara Starfield and Lisa Simpson, "Primary Care as Part of the U.S. Health Services Reform," *JAMA* 269 (1993): 3136–39.

44 Howard Wolinsky, "Fed Up With Hassles and Financial Woes, Some General Internists Quit Their Practices," *ACP Observer* 12 (992): 10.

44 Jeanne Kassler, "Managed Care—or Chaos?" *New York Magazine,* August 23, 1993: 44–50.

45 Daniel Berstein, "Medical Student and Choice of Speciality," (letter) *JAMA* 267 (1992): 1921.

45 Robert Petersdorf, "Primary Care Applicants—They Get No Respect," *New England Journal of Medicine* 326 (1992): 408–9.

46 Sheldon Greenfield et al., "Variations in Resource Utilization Among Medical Specialties and Systems of Care," *JAMA* 267 (1992): 1624–30.

Chapter 5: Privacy—Threatened by Computers and Commerce

48 Mubarak Dahir, "Your Health, Your Privacy, Your Boss," Philadelphia City Paper, May 28–June 4, 1993: 10–11.

49 Michael Miller, "Congress, AMA Move to Protect Patient Records," *Wall Street Journal,* July 10, 1992: B2.

49 Michael Miller, "Patients' Records Are Treasure Trove for Budding Industry," *Wall Street Journal,* February 27, 1992: A1.

49 "National Crime Information Center," testimony by Laurie Ekstrand, July 28, 1993, GAO/T-GGD-93-41: 5.

50 "National Crime Information Center," testimony by Laurie Ekstrand, July 28, 1993, GAO/T-GGD-93-41: 6–7, 16.

50 "Healthcare Network Forms," *New York Times,* September 8, 1993: D13.

50 Protecting Privacy in Computerized Medical Information. Office of Technology Assessment. September, 1993: 16–17, 26.

50 Rhonda Vincent, assistant VP of investor relations, personal communication.

51 Sharon McIlrath, "Bush Says Plan Cuts Health Care Hassles," *American Medical News,* June 29, 1992: 1.

51 Greg Borzo, "Ready or Not, EDI Is Coming," *American Medical News,* July 12, 1993: 2.

52 Gabriella Stern, "P&G Keeps Tabs on Workers, Others, New Book Asserts." *Wall Street Journal,* September 7, 1993: A3.

52 Stephanie Strom, "K Mart Is Sued by 43 Workers in Privacy Case in Illinois," *New York Times,* September 15, 1993: D5.

52 WEDI news release, November 23, 1993.

52 Mary Carnevale, "Caller ID Services Accused of Invading Individuals' Privacy," *Wall Street Journal,* June 25, 1993: B2.

53 "Johnson & Johnson Respondents Offered," *DM News,* June 21, 1993: 2.

53 Ralph Larsen to Edward J. Markey, July 7, 1993.

53 Mary Darby, "Pharmaceutical Firms Explore New Tactic: Building Lifelong Relationships With Patients," *ACP Observer* 12 (September 1992): 1.

54 Michael Miller, "Patients' Records Are Treasure Trove for Budding Industry," *Wall Street Journal,* February 27, 1992: A1.

54 Sara Calian, "Medical Marketing's Prospects Are Said to Be Clouded by Possible Competition," *Wall Street Journal*, August 24, 1992: C6.
54 "McKesson Corp. Unit Contract," *Wall Street Journal*, February 10, 1993: B5.
54 Blair Jackson, VP corporate communications, PCS Health Systems, Inc., personal communication, September 27, 1993.
54 Personal communication (fax), October 4, 1993.
55 Ron Winslow and Hilary Stout, "Insurers Select McKesson Unit to Speed Claims," *Wall Street Journal*, July 22, 1992: B1.
55 Michael Quint, "Primerica in Talks to Create a Financial Giant," *New York Times*, September 23, 1993: D1.
55 George Anders, "Medco's Sale Holds Fee of $60 Million for Chief Wygod," *Wall Street Journal*, July 30, 1993: B5.
55 Elyse Tanouye, "Merck Will Exploit Medco's Database," *Wall Street Journal*, August 4, 1993: B1.
56 Physician Computer Network, Inc., Annual Report, 1991.
57 Physician Computer Network, Inc., Form 10-K, 1991: 8.
57 Michael Miller, "Patients' Records Are Treasure Trove for Budding Industry," *Wall Street Journal*, February 27, 1992: A1.
58 MIB, Inc.: "A Consumer's Guide," and personal communication.
58 Andrea Adelson, "Transamerica Draws Fire on Cancer Test," *New York Times*, April 24, 1993: 36.
59 Mubarak Dahir, "Your Health, Your Privacy, Your Boss," Philadelphia City Paper, May 28–June 24, 1993: 10–11.
59 Julia Interrante, Genzyme Public Relations, personal communication, November 18, 1993.

Chapter 6: The Booming New Industries of Health Care

65 Simon Francis, "U.S. Industrial Outlook 1993—Health and Medical Services," U.S. Commerce Department: 42–44.
65 *Wall Street Journal*, April 4, 1993: B3.
66 Investment Analysis, Needham & Co., January 24, 1992.
66 Timothy O'Brien, "Curaflex Zeroes In on a Niche to Succeed in Home Care," *Wall Street Journal*, August 5, 1992: B2.
66 *Grace News*, May 19, 1993, and July 19, 1993.
66 T² Medical, Inc., 10-K filing, 1993: 1.
66 David Stipp, "Blue Cross Plan for Home-Infusion Upheld in Boston," *Wall Street Journal*, July 22, 1992: C11.
67 Timothy O'Brien, "Curaflex Zeroes on a Niche to Succeed in Home Care," *Wall Street Journal*, August 5, 1992: B2.
67 Andrea Gerlin, "Lyme Disease Spurs Disputes Over Treatment," *Wall Street Journal*, July 28, 1992: B1.
67 Investment Analysis, Needham & Co., January 24, 1992.
67 T² Medical, 1991 Annual Report: 1.
67 Karen Rak, "T² and Tokos Medical Launch Women's Homecare, Inc.," *Home Health Line*, July 10, 1991.
67 T² news release, May 11, 1992.
67 Jerry Schwartz, "T² Medical Stock Plunges; Two Executives Step Down," *New York Times*, August 13, 1993: D1.
67 Emory Thomas, Jr., "Managers' Plan to Buy T² Collapses, and Company's Shares Tumble 15%," *Wall Street Journal*, September 9, 1993: A6.
68 George Anders, "Rx for Sales," *Wall Street Journal*, September 10, 1993: A1.

68 Medical Marketing Group, Inc., "First Defectors," 1991.

68 Medical Marketing Group, Inc., "Patient Direct," 1991.

69 George Anders, "Medco Hires Ex-President of Citicorp," *Wall Street Journal*, December 9, 1992: B10.

69 Physician *Micro*marketing Incorporated, "Physician Psychological Profiling."

69 F-D-C Reports (The "Pink Sheet"), May 11, 1992: 7–9.

70 "Medical Marketing Group, Inc.," *Wall Street Journal*, November 17, 1993: B14.

70 Karen Davis, "Controlling Health Care Expenditures: Expenditure Limits and Managed Competition," remarks for roundtable discussion at Columbia University, February 8, 1993.

71 George Anders, "Battle of HMOs for Military Job Could Be Model," *Wall Street Journal*, July 8, 1993: B1.

71 Tom Morganthau and Andrew Murr, "Inside the World of an HMO," *Newsweek*, April 5, 1993: 34–40.

71 "HMO Contract Dispute," *Wall Street Journal*, January 6, 1993: B6.

72 Ron Winslow, "U.S. Healthcare Says Earnings Advanced 63%," *Wall Street Journal*, October 26, 1993: B6.

72 PacifiCare Health Systems, Inc., 1991 Annual Report: 2.

72 Foundation Health Corporation, 1991 Annual Report: 2.

72 Karen Davis, "Controlling Health Care Expenditures: Expenditure Limits and Managed Competition," remarks for roundtable discussion at Columbia University, February 8, 1993.

72 Vernon Staines, "Potential Impact of Managed Care on National Health Spending," *Health Affairs*, Supplement 1993: 253.

73 "The Effects of Managed Care on Use and Costs of Health Services," CBO staff memorandum, June 1992: 7, 16.

73 "U.S. Health Care Spending," General Accounting Office, GAO/HRD-91-102, June 1991: 15.

73 "U.S. Healthcare's New York Request on Rates Is Rejected," *Wall Street Journal*, January 2, 1992: A14.

73 U.S. Healthcare, Annual Report, 1991: 35–36.

73 PacifiCare Health Systems, Inc., 1991 Annual Report: 24.

74 Foundation Health Corporation, 1991 Annual Report: 18–19.

74 Jeanne Kassler, "Managed Care—or Chaos?" *New York Magazine*, August 23, 1993: 44–50.

74 Milt Freundenheim, "New Ways to Help Injured Workers," *New York Times*, October 27, 1992: D2.

75 "HMO America Stock Off 14%," *New York Times*, May 14, 1992: D5.

75 Alan Hillman, "Health Maintenance Organizations, Financial Incentives, and Physicians' Judgments," *Annals of Internal Medicine* 112 (1990): 891–93.

76 Allan Brett, "The Case Against Persuasive Advertising by Health Maintenance Organizations," *New England Journal of Medicine* 326 (1992): 1353–56.

76 Asha Wallace, "HMOs and Physicians Without Board Certification," *New England Journal of Medicine* (letter), 328 (1993): 1501–2.

77 Milt Freudenheim, "2 Largest Hospital Chains in U.S. Agree to Merge," *New York Times*, October 3, 1993: 25.

77 Arnold Relman, "Investor-Owned Hospitals and Health-Care Costs," *New England Journal of Medicine* 309 (1983): 370–72.

78 Greg Donaldson, director of corporate communications, Humana, personal communication, September 23, 1993.

78 "Humana Cuts Jobs; Sets Up 3 Companies," *New York Times*, August 18, 1992: D4.

78 Jeffrey Birnbaum, "Humana Reported Improper Medicare Costs, US Says," *Wall Street Journal*, June 12, 1992: A6.

78 Advertisement in *Wall Street Journal*, June 26, 1992.

78 Humana Inc., *Value Line*, November 6, 1992: 1280.

79 Ron Winslow, "Experts Try to Gauge Mental-Health Care," *Wall Street Journal*, December 1, 1992: B1.

79 Rhonda Rundle, "Rehabilitation Facilities Brace for Texas Investigation," *Wall Street Journal*, June 16, 1992: B4.

79 "Nat'l Med. Ent.," *Value Line*, November 6, 1992: 1282.

79 Thomas King, "Hospital Firm to Restructure Troubled Unit," *Wall Street Journal*, April 24, 1992: A8.

79 Sonia Nazario, "Allegations of Fraud, Malpractice Still Haunt Operator of Hospitals," *Wall Street Journal*, January 8, 1993: A1.

80 Insider Trading Spotlight, *Wall Street Journal*, May 19, 1993: B4.

80 Rhonda Rundle, "National Medical Enterprises Relieves Co-Founder Bedrosian of His Duties," *Wall Street Journal*, September 27, 1993: B10.

80 Rhonda Rundle, "National Medical Agrees to Changes, Settles Texas Suit," *Wall Street Journal*, June 4, 1992: B9.

80 Peter Kerr, "Mental Hospital Operator Settles Lawsuit with Texas," *New York Times*, June 5, 1992: D6.

80 Sonia Nazario, "Allegations of Fraud, Malpractice Still Haunt Operator of Hospitals," *Wall Street Journal*, January 8, 1993: A1.

80 Peter Kerr, "8 Insurers Sue National Medical Enterprises," *New York Times*, July 31, 1992: D1.

80 Rhonda Rundle, "National Medical Discloses Probe of Two Hospitals," *Wall Street Journal*, April 15, 1993: B6.

80 Rhonda Rundle, "National Medical Facilities Raided by U.S. Agents," *Wall Street Journal*, August 27, 1993: A3.

80 Rhonda Rundle, "National Medical Agrees to Payment of $89.9 Million to Settle Insurance Suit," *Wall Street Journal*, December 14, 1993: A4.

80 Helene Cooper, "Charter Medical Sells Surgical Hospitals in Move to Focus on Psychiatric Business," *Wall Street Journal*, August 10, 1993: A3.

80 Daniel Pearl, "Charter Medical Agrees to Reforms at Texas Hospitals," *Wall Street Journal*, January 4, 1993: B2.

80 Peter Kerr, "Treating of Severe Brain Injuries Is Profitable, but Not for Patients," *New York Times*, March 16, 1992: A1.

80 Rhonda Rundle, "Rehabilitation Facilities Brace for Texas Investigation," *Wall Street Journal*, June 16, 1992: B4.

80 Ron Suskind, "Head-Trauma Firm's Records Seized by Federal Agents in Fraud Inquiry," *Wall Street Journal*, October 28, 1992: A6.

81 Peter Kerr, "Treating of Severe Brain Injuries Is Profitable, but Not for Patients," *New York Times*, March 16, 1992: A1.

81 Rhonda Rundle, "Rehabilitation Facilities Brace for Texas Investigation," *Wall Street Journal*, June 16, 1992: B4.

81 "Integrated Health Cites Increased Profit on Continuing Lines," *Wall Street Journal*, July 7, 1992: B4C.

81 Robert Tomsho, "Limited-Service Hospitals Find a Market," *Wall Street Journal*, July 23, 1992: B1.

82 Milt Freudenheim, "2 Largest Hospital Chains in U.S. Agree to Merge," *New York Times,* October 3, 1993: 25.

82 Bob Ortega, "Columbia Joins Medical Care in Affiliate Pact," *Wall Street Journal,* October 8, 1993: A3.

82 Robert Tomsho, "A Wunderkind Who's Gobbling Hospital Chains," *Wall Street Journal,* October 5, 1993: B1.

82 Randall Smith, "Player in HCA-Columbia Merger Sees Combination as Wal-Mart of Health," *Wall Street Journal,* October 4, 1993: A6.

83 Arnold Relman, "The New Medical-Industrial Complex," *New England Journal of Medicine* 303 (1980): 963–700.

83 John Iglehart, "The End Stage Renal Disease Program," *New England Journal of Medicine* 328 (1993): 366–71.

83 Physician Payment Review Commission, Annual Report to Congress, 1989: 8.

83 Health Care Financing Administration, Research Report, "End Stage Renal Disease, 1990": 63.

84 Health Care Financing Administration, "End Stage Renal Disease Patient Pacific Profile Tables 1991": 2.

84 Health Care Financing Administration, Research Report, "End Stage Renal Disease, 1990": 3–4, 53.

84 Richard Kusserow, "The Red Book: 1992 Office of Inspector General Cost-Saver Handbook," HCFA: J1.

84 Gina Kolata, "NMC Thrives Selling Dialysis," *Science* 208 (1980): 379–82.

84 *Wall Street Journal,* April 14, 1993: B11.

85 Gina Kolata, "NMC Thrives Selling Dialysis," *Science* 208 (1980): 379–82.

85 "Reductions Continue to Be Needed in Medicare's End Stage Renal Dialysis Rates," Office of Inspector General, July 16, 1990, Report A-14-90-00215.

86 *United States Department of Commerce News,* April 9, 1993.

86 HHS news release, September 14, 1992.

86 Helene Cooper, "REN to Expand Dialysis Units Over 3 Years," *Wall Street Journal,* October 5, 1992: A7C.

86 Glenn Kramon, "Infertility Chain: The Good and Bad in Medicine," *New York Times,* June 19, 1992: D1.

86 Alison Cowan, "Can a Baby-Making Venture Deliver?" *New York Times,* June 1, 1992: D1.

87 IVF America, Prospectus, October 8, 1992: 18.

88 Suzanne Alexander, "American Medical Response Says Net Almost Doubled in the Second Quarter," *Wall Street Journal,* September 14, 1992: B9G.

88 "Premier Anesthesia Says Earnings Soared in Second Quarter," *Wall Street Journal,* July 20, 1992: B3C.

88 "Premier Anesthesia," *Wall Street Journal,* August 23, 1993: B3.

88 Thomas Burton, "Firms That Promise Lower Medical Bills May Increase Them," *Wall Street Journal,* July 28, 1992: A1.

88 "Employers Say They're in the Dark on Effects of Utilization Review," *Medical Utilization Review,* April 16, 1992: 2.

89 Thomas Burton, "Firms That Promise Lower Medical Bills May Increase Them," *Wall Street Journal,* July 28, 1992: A1.

89 Linda Oberman, "Can an Accreditation System Take the Irritation Out of Utilization Review?" *American Medical News,* October 2, 1992: 3.

89 "Utilization Review," General Accounting Office, GAO/HRD-93-22FS, November 1992: 55–56.

90 Thomas Burton, "Firms That Promise Lower Medical Bills May Increase Them," *Wall Street Journal,* July 28, 1992: A1.

91 David Azevedo, "Courts Let UR Firms Off the Hook—and Leave Doctors On," *Medical Economics,* January 25, 1993: 30–44.

91 Edward Felsenthal and Milo Geyelin, "Courts Support Health Insurers That Reject 'Unnecessary' Care," *Wall Street Journal,* November 25, 1992: B8.

Chapter 7: The Pharmaceutical Industry

94 American Society of Internal Medicine report, "The Rising Costs of Prescription Drugs," June 23, 1992: 3, 5.

94 Elyse Tanouye, "Drug Companies Post Sales Gains for 2nd Quarter," *Wall Street Journal,* July 21, 1992: C21.

94 Elyse Tanouye, "Drug Makers Likely to Show Slim Profit Rise," *Wall Street Journal,* July 12, 1993: B7A.

94 Karl Kimbel, "Germany: One-Sided Prescription Boom," *Lancet* 340 (1992): 903.

95 Jonathan Edelson, "Long-term Cost-Effectiveness of Various Initial Monotherapies for Mild to Moderate Hypertension," *JAMA* 263 (1990): 407–13.

95 Marilyn Chase, "Doctor Assails J&J Price Tag on Cancer Drug," *Wall Street Journal,* May 20, 1992: B1.

95 Cancer Patient Sues Johnson & Johnson Over Drug Pricing," *Wall Street Journal,* August 18, 1992: B6.

95 Michael Waldholz, "Cost May Limit Use of Pfizer Drug Against Chlamydia," *Wall Street Journal,* September 24, 1992: B3.

95 Daniel Bross, "The Dark Side of Astra: High Prices on AIDS Drug" (letter), *New York Times,* December 27, 1992: F11.

95 Elyse Tanouye, "Norplant's Maker Draws Sharp Criticism on Pricing of Long-Acting Contraceptive," *Wall Street Journal,* August 30, 1993: B1.

95 Elyse Tanouye, "Estrogen Drug Revives American Home Products Sales," *Wall Street Journal,* August 10, 1992: B4.

96 Milt Freundenheim, "Canadians See Rise in Drug Costs," *New York Times,* November 16, 1992: D1.

96 Milt Freundenheim, "Canadian Drug-Price Shift Said to Cost $3.2 Billion," *New York Times,* December 1, 1992: D6.

96 John Iglehart, "The American Health Care System: Medicaid," *New England Journal of Medicine* 328 (1993): 896–900.

96 Milt Freundenheim, "Tax Credits of $8.5 Billion Received by 22 Drug Makers," *New York Times,* May 15, 1992: D3.

96 Hilary Stout, "Drug Firms Get Tax Break Exceeding $70,90 for Each Worker in Puerto Rico," *Wall Street Journal,* May 15, 1992: A4.

97 Clifford Krauss, "Legislators to Restore Tax Breaks to U.S. Companies in Puerto Rico," *New York Times,* July 24, 1993: 26.

97 "IRS Ruling Will Benefit Multinational Companies," *Wall Street Journal,* June 25, 1992: B2.

97 Suzanne Tregarthen, "Prescription to Stop Drug Companies' Profiteering," *Wall Street Journal,* March 5, 1992: A15 (op-ed).

97 Philip Hilts, "Seeking Limits to a Drug Monopoly," *New York Times,* May 14, 1992: D1.

97 Office of Inspector General, Semi-Annual Report, October 1, 1990–March 1, 1992: 25.

98 David Stipp, " 'Gene Therapy' for Gaucher's Disease Shows Promising Results in Test on Mice," *Wall Street Journal,* December 3, 1992: B6.

98 Philip Hilts, "Seeking Limits to a Drug Monopoly," *New York Times,* May 14, 1992: D1.

98 Suzanne Tregarthen, "Prescription to Stop Drug Companies' Profiteering," *Wall Street Journal,* March 5, 1992: A15 (op-ed).

98 "Questions Arise Over Price of Bristol-Myers's Taxol," *Wall Street Journal,* October 26, 1992: B2.

98 Elyse Tanouye, "Bristol-Myers Plans to Seek Approval to Market Taxol," *Wall Street Journal,* March 5, 1992: B6.

98 Michael Waldholz, "Specter of Regulation Sets Off Price War," *Wall Street Journal,* September 25, 1992: A4.

99 Robert Pear, "Drug Industry Musters a Coalition to Oppose a Change in Medicaid," *New York Times,* July 7, 1993: A1.

99 VA News Service.

99 Michael Wilkes et al., "Pharmaceutical Advertisements in Leading Medical Journals: Experts' Assessments," *Annals of Internal Medicine* 116 (1992): 912–19.

99 Joanne Lipman, "List of Offending Drug Advertisers May Lead to Crackdown by FDA," *Wall Street Journal,* July 31, 1992: B5.

100 Robert Fletcher and Suzanne Fletcher, "Pharmaceutical Advertising in Medical Journals," *Annals of Internal Medicine* 116 (1992): 951–52.

100 Lisa Bero et al., "The Publication of Sponsored Symposiums in Medical Journals," *New England Journal of Medicine* 327 (1992): 1135–40.

100 Mike Mitka, "Drug Firm Events Linked to Changes in Prescribing Habits," *American Medical News,* May 25, 1992: 29.

101 John Emery, American Business Press, personal communication.

101 Elyse Tanouye, "Nicotine Patch Promotion Blitz Draws Scrutiny," *Wall Street Journal,* October 19, 1992: B1.

101 Michael Waldholz, "Merck May Face Problems in Sale of Prostate Drug," *Wall Street Journal,* June 23, 1992: B6.

101 Merck advertisement, *New York Times,* November 9, 1992: A5.

102 Jane Brody, "Nationwide Tests Set for Prostate Cancer, but Doubts Surface," *New York Times,* September 20, 1992: A1.

102 Elyse Tanouye, "Drug Firms Start 'Compliance' Programs Reminding Patients to Take Their Pills," *Wall Street Journal,* March 25, 1992: B1.

Chapter 8: The Medical Profession

104 Robert Blendon, "The Public View of Medicine" (from a lecture at the 39th Congress of Neurological Surgeons), *Clinical Neurosurgery* (Baltimore: Williams & Wilkins, 1989), 225–31.

105 Ron Winslow, "U.S. Doctors Express Least Satisfaction in Three-Nation Survey of Health Care," *Wall Street Journal,* June 9, 1992: B5.

105 *Wall Street Journal,* December 22, 1992: A1.

105 Jack Colwill, "Where Have All the Primary Care Applicants Gone?" *New England Journal of Medicine* 326 (1992): 387–93.

106 Howard Larkin, "Employee Doctor Pay Found Comparable to Private Practice," *American Medical News,* July 20, 1992: 21.

106 William Hsiao et al., "Assessing the Implementation of the Physician-Payment Reform," *New England Journal of Medicine* 328 (1993): 928–33.

107 Health and Human Services news release, May 7, 1993.

107 Louis Harris and Associates, "Physicians and Medicare Fee Schedule: A Look at the Medicare Program and Other Payers in a Changing Practice Environment," February 1993: 32–33.

107 William Hsiao, "RBRVS: Objections to Maloney, 1," *JAMA* 267 (1992): 1822–23.

107 "Surgeons Paid More—Even by Pollsters," *American Medical News*, October 12, 1992: 7.

107 Physician Payment Review Commission, Annual Report to Congress, 1993: 129–30.

107 Louis Harris and Associates, "Physicians and Medicare Fee Schedule: A Look at the Medicare Program and Other Payers in a Changing Practice Environment," February 1993: 6, 8.

108 Barry Stimmel, "The Crisis in Primary Care and the Role of Medical Schools," *JAMA* 268 (1992): 2060–65.

109 Howard Larkin, "Overhead Expenses Are on the Rise," *American Medical News*, March 23/30, 1992: 21.

110 Arnold Relman, " 'Self-Referral'—What's at Stake?" *New England Journal of Medicine* 327 (1992): 1522–24.

111 Robert Blendon, "The Public View of Medicine" (from a lecture at the 39th Congress of Neurological Surgeons), *Clinical Neurosurgery* (Baltimore: Williams & Wilkins, 1989): 225–31.

111 Arnold Relman, "The New Medical-Industrial Complex," *New England Journal of Medicine* 303 (1980): 963–700.

112 Jeanne Kassler, "Managed Care—or Chaos?" *New York Magazine*, August 23, 1993: 48.

113 "Medicaid. HealthPASS: An Evaluation of a Managed Care Program for Certain Philadelphia Recipients," General Accounting Office, GAO/HRD-93-67, May 1993: 15, 36.

113 Felicity Barringer, "Hospital Executives' Pay Rose Sharply in Decade," *New York Times*, September 9, 1992: A14.

Chapter 9: The Media

116 "Investigations of Patients Who Have Been Treated for HIV-Infected Health-Care Workers," *Morbidity and Mortality Weekly Report* 41 (1992): 344–460.

117 Lawrence Altman, "Study Sees No New Transmissions of H.I.V. by Health-Care Workers," *New York Times*, March 15, 1992: A18.

117 William Hsiao et al., "Assessing the Implementation of Physician-Payment Reform," *New England Journal of Medicine* 328 (1993): 928–33.

118 William Roper, "The Resource-Based Relative Value Scale: A Methodological and Policy Evaluation," *JAMA* 260 (1988): 2444–46.

118 Philip Hilts, "Doctors' Pay Underestimated but Resented Just the Same," *New York Times*, March 31, 1993: A21.

118 Joseph Belth, *The Insurance Forum*, August 1993.

119 Natalie Angier, "Scientists Report Novel Therapy for Brain Tumors," *New York Times*, June 12, 1992: D17.

119 David Stipp, "New Device Set to Eliminate Kidney Stones," *Wall Street Journal*, June 4, 1991: B4.

119 "New Test May Spot Metastasis of Cancer to Bones," *New York Times*, August 4, 1992: C3.

119 Robert Calem, "New Guards Against Infection," *New York Times*, July 7, 1992: F9.

120 Michael Specter, "Neglected for Years, TB Is Back With Strains That Are Deadlier," *New York Times*, October 11, 1992: A1.
120 Jeanne Kassler, "Drug-Resistant Tuberculosis Is Surging," *New York Times*, June 2, 1992: LI1.
121 Lawrence Altman, "Terminally Ill Man Gets Baboon's Liver in Untried Operation," *New York Times*, June 29, 1992: A1.
121 *New York Times*, January 10, 1993: A1.
121 Lawrence Altman, "Recipient of Liver Dies After Stroke," *New York Times*, September 8, 1992: D14.
121 Natalie Angier, "With Direct Injections, Gene Therapy Takes a Step Into a New Age," *New York Times*, April 14, 1992: C3.
121 "Teen-Agers and AIDS: The Risk Worsens," *New York Times*, April 14, 1992: C3.
122 Gary Schwitzer, "The Magical Medical Media Tour," *JAMA* 267 (1992): 1969–71.
123 Gary Schwitzer, "The Magical Medical Media Tour," *JAMA* 267 (1992): 1969–71.
123 Morton Mintz, "Veteran Reporter Finds New Target: Outside Directors," *Newsletter of National Association of Science Writers* 39 (1992): 3–6.
124 Laura Bird, "Corporate Critics Complain Companies Hide Behind 'Grass-Roots' Campaigns," *Wall Street Journal*, July 8, 1992: B1.
124 Kevin Goldman, "Cancer Society Runs Ad Ideas Past Media," *Wall Street Journal*, December 16, 1992: B10.
125 Morton Mintz, "Veteran Reporter Finds New Target: Outside Directors," *Newsletter of National Association of Science Writers* 39 (1992): 3–6.
125 Brandon Centerwall, "Television and Violence, *JAMA* 267 (1992): 3059–63.
125 Edmund Andrews, "4 Networks Agree to Offer Warnings of Violence on TV," *New York Times*, June 30, 1993: A1.
125 Bob Herbert, "Violence in Real Life," *New York Times*, July 11, 1993: E19.
125 Lisa Belkin, "In Lessons on Empathy, Doctors Become Patients," *New York Times*, June 4, 1992: A1.
126 Natalie Angier, "Bedside Manners Improve as More Women Enter Medicine," *New York Times*, June 21, 1992: IV 18.
126 Nina Sandlin, "Seeing the Rainbow," *American Medical News*, January 4, 1993: 3.

Chapter 10: American Values—
A Backdrop for Health Care and Its Reform

128 Times Mirror Center for the People and the Press, "The Public, Their Doctors, and Health Care Reform," April 14, 1992.
129 Robert Blendon et al., "Bridging the Gap Between Expert and Public Views on Health Care Reform," *JAMA* 1993: 2573–78.
129 Natalie Angier, "Many Americans Say Genetic Information Is Public Property," *New York Times*, September 29, 1992: C2.
130 Robert Blendon et al., "Physicians' Perspectives on Caring for Patients in the United States, Canada, and West Germany," *New England Journal of Medicine* 328 (1993): 1011–16.
130 David Eddy, "Three Battles to Watch in the 1990s," *JAMA* 270 (1993): 520–526.
130 "As Quadruplets Hang On, a Welfare Fight Rages," *New York Times*, March 29, 1992: A21.

130 Deborah Mesce, "Plans to Open VA Hospitals in Ala., Va. to Non-Vets Canceled," AP, February 21, 1992.

131 Eliot Marshall, "The Politics of Breast Cancer," *Science* 259 (1993): 616–17.

131 James Weaver, "The Best Care Other People's Money Can Buy," *Wall Street Journal,* November 19, 1992: A14 (op-ed).

131 Physician Payment Review Commission, Annual Report to Congress, 1989: 22.

132 George Annas, "Adding Injustice to Injury: Compulsory Payment for Unwanted Treatment," *New England Journal of Medicine* 327 (1992): 1885–87.

Chapter 11: Government

135 Health and Human Services news release, March 17, 1993.

135 John Iglehart, "The American Health Care System—Medicaid," *New England Journal of Medicine* 328 (1993): 896–900.

135 George Anders, "Health-Care Fund Fight Erupts Over States' Use of the Federal 'Disproportionate Share' Clause," *Wall Street Journal,* June 3, 1993: A16.

136 "New Jersey Seeking New Ways to Provide Indigent Health Care," *Wall Street Journal,* May 29, 1992: A5.

136 James Dao, "Deal Made to Save New York Hospital Surcharge," *New York Times,* August 4, 1993: B7.

136 Health and Human Services news release, April 2, 1992.

136 Robert Pear, "Audit of Government Says Billions Are Being Wasted," *New York Times,* January 8, 1993: A10.

137 Health Care Financing Administration, fact sheet, January 1993.

137 The Medicare 1992 Handbook, U.S. Department of Health and Human Services: 1.

137 "Retirees of Exempt Government Agencies Are a Financial Drain of Medicare Part A Funds," DHHS Office of Inspector General Memorandum, February 23, 1989.

138 U.S. General Accounting Office, "Health and Human Services Issues," December 1992: 4.

138 U.S. General Accounting Office, "Medicare Claims," December 1992.

138 Congressional Budget Office, "Economic Implications of Rising Health Care Costs," October 1992: 49.

138 John Iglehart, "The American Health Care System: Medicare," *New England Journal of Medicine* 327 (1992): 1467–72.

138 Robert Pear, "Audit of Government Says Billions Are Being Wasted," *New York Times,* January 8, 1993: A10.

138 Steven Holmes, "Federal Contracts Gave Perot His Big Break," *New York Times,* June 5, 1992: A1.

139 "Final Results: Medicare Influenza Vaccine Demonstration," *Morbidity and Mortality Weekly Report* 42 (1993): 601–4.

139 Health and Human Services news release, November 20, 1992.

140 William Hsiao et al., "Assessing the Implementation of Physician-Payment Reform," *New England Journal of Medicine* 328 (1993): 928–33.

140 Elizabeth Neus, "Employers, Labor Unite to Oppose Benefits Tax," *Chicago Sun-Times,* February 10, 1993: 21.

141 Simon Francis, "U.S. Industrial Outlook 1993—Health and Medical Services," U.S. Commerce Department: 42–44.

141 Paul Starr and Walter Zelman, "A Bridge to Compromise: Competition Under a Budget," *Health Affairs Supplement,* 1993: 18.

141 John Dingell, "Misconduct in Medical Research," *New England Journal of Medicine* 328 (1993): 1610–15.

141 Philip Hilts, "Congress Urged to Lift Ban on Fetal-Tissue Research," *New York Times*, May 27, 1992: A12.

142 Philip Hilts, "Fetal-Tissue Bank Cannot Meet Goal, Agency Memo Says," *New York Times*, July 27, 1992: A1.

142 Elyse Tanouye, "Abortion-Rights Forces Plan to Pursue Return of Pills Despite Justices' Ruling," *Wall Street Journal*, July 20, 1992: B6.

142 "Key Lobbyist Wins AIDS Vaccine Trials," *New York Times*, October 20, 1992: C2.

143 Marilyn Chase and Thomas Ricks, "U.S. to Test MicroGeneSys AIDS Vaccine After Firm Torpedoes Broader Study," *Wall Street Journal*, August 23, 1993: B3.

143 Barry Meier, "Scientists Assail Congress on Bill for Money to Test an AIDS Drug," *New York Times*, October 26, 1992: A1.

143 Vicki Kemper and Viveca Novak, "A Plague on Both Their Houses," *Common Cause Magazine*, October 1992: 2.

144 Michael Wines, "Candidates for Congress Spent Record $678 Million, a 52% Jump," *New York Times*, March 5, 1993: A12.

144 Robert Pear, "Conflicting Aims in Booming Health Care Lobby Help Stall Congress," *New York Times*, March 18, 1992: A17.

144 Vicki Kemper and Viveca Novak, "A Plague on Both Their Houses," *Common Cause Magazine*, October 1991: 1–8.

144 "Health and Insurance PAC's Political Gifts Rose 22%, Group Says," *Wall Street Journal*, July 23, 1992: A14.

144 "Health Care Industry Funnels Money to Senator Wofford," *American Medical News*, March 1, 1993: 20.

144 Larry Mackinson, *"The Cash Constituents of Congress,"* Center for Responsive Politics, 1992: 73.

144 Clifford Krauss, "Lawmakers' Legal Aid Society: Rich Donors," *New York Times*, August 13, 1993: B7.

145 Josh Goldstein, Center for Responsive Politics, personal communication, September 28, 1993.

145 "Gradison to Take HIAA Post; Thomas Fills Ways & Means Seat," *Medicine and Health*, January 11, 1993: 3.

146 Matthew Wald, "Experts Say Fear of Asbestos Exceeds the Risk in Schools," *New York Times*, September 4, 1993: A1.

146 Selwyn Raab, "School Asbestos Inquiry Is Focusing on Choice of Labs by Contractor," *New York Times*, August 15, 1993: 39.

146 William Rutala and David Weber, "Infectious Waste—Mismatch Between Science and Policy," *New England Journal of Medicine* 325 (1992): 578–81.

147 William Rutala and David Weber, "Infectious Waste—Mismatch Between Science and Policy," *New England Journal of Medicine* 325 (1992): 578–81.

147 Diane Gianelli, "Gentler Lab Regulations," *American Medical News*, September 14, 1992: 1.

147 Charles Marwick and Phil Gunby, "Clinical Laboratory Improvement Amendments Finally May Go Into Effect September 1," *JAMA* 267 (1992): 1441.

147 Calvin Sims, "Blood Labs Agree to Pay $39.8 Million," *New York Times*, September 14, 1993: D1.

147 Milt Freudenheim, "U.S. Subpoenas Blood-Test Files in New Health Care Fraud Inquiry," *New York Times*, August 8, 1993: A1.

147 Julie Johnsson, "New Medicaid Drug Rules: Better Care, More Hassle," *American Medical News*, December 7, 1992: 10.

148 Occupational Safety and Health Administration, public information specialist.

148 "Medical-Apparel Rule Is Boon for Laundries," *Wall Street Journal*, August 14, 1992: B1.

148 Jonathan Weil, "Federal Regulations to Prevent Infection of Health-Care Workers Will Be Costly," *Wall Street Journal*, July 2, 1992: B1.

148 Martha Goldsmith, "OSHA Bloodborne Pathogens Standard Aims to Limit Occupational Transmission," *JAMA* 267 (1992): 2853–54.

148 George Anders, "Hospital Administrative Costs Surge as Regulatory Requirements Increase," *Wall Street Journal*, July 1, 1993: B6.

149 John Iglehart, "The End Stage Renal Disease Program," *New England Journal of Medicine* 328 (1993): 366–71.

149 Hilary Stout, "More Than 100 Hospitals Had High Death Rates in 1990," *Wall Street Journal*, June 11, 1992: B8.

149 "Mortality Data on Medicare-Test Hospital," *Wall Street Journal*, June 11, 1992: B8.

151 Ellen Shapiro, "Health Group Seeks Tobacco Tax Rise to Generate Revenue, Reduce Smoking," *Wall Street Journal*, January 5, 1993: A6B.

151 Suein Hwang, "Philip Morris Posts Net of $1.1 Billion for the 1st Quarter," *Wall Street Journal*, April 17, 1992: A3.

151 "Update Tobacco: Healthy for the Economy?" *American Medical News*, June 22, 1992: 17.

151 Charles Culhane, "Tobacco Industry Gave Millions to Political Parties," *American Medical News*, September 14, 1992: 11.

151 Eben Shapiro, "Health Group Seeks Tobacco Tax Rise to Generate Revenue, Reduce Smoking," *Wall Street Journal*, January 5, 1993: A6B.

151 "Smoking Among Adults," *Morbidity and Mortality Weekly Report* 41 (1992): 360–62.

152 Paul Cotton, "Gun-Associated Violence Increasingly Viewed as Public Health Challenge," *JAMA* 267 (1992): 1171–73.

152 Marsha Goldsmith, " 'Invisible' Epidemic Now Becoming Visible as HIV/AIDS Epidemic Reaches Adolescents," *JAMA* 270 (1993): 16–19.

152 Finnish embassy, pesonal communication.

153 David Kirp and Ronald Bayer, "Needles and Race," *Atlantic*, July 1993: 38–42.

153 Robert Pear, "Arkansas Struggles to Deal With Rising Health-Care Costs for the Poor," *New York Times*, October 19, 1992: A12.

153 Timothy Egan, "Oregon Seeks to Revive Health Care 'Rationing' Plan," *New York Times*, August 14, 1992.

153 Robert Pear, "Too-Bitter Medicine," *New York Times*, August 5, 1992: A14.

154 Fox Butterfield, "Universal Health Care Plan Is Goal of Law in Vermont," *New York Times*, May 12, 1992: A12.

154 Barbara Yawn et al., "MinnesotaCare (HealthRight)—Myths and Miracles," *JAMA* 269 (1993): 511–15.

154 "Minnesota Law Faces ERISA Challenge," *Medicine & Health*, September 14, 1992: 2.

Chapter 12: Malpractice and the Legal System

155 Wendy Parmet, "The Impact of Health Insurance Reform on the Law Governing the Physician-Patient Relationship," *JAMA* 268 (1992): 2468–72.

155 Edward Wrobel, Jr., "Out of Remission," *Emphasis* 4 (1992): 6–9.

155 "Medical Malpractice: Experience With Efforts to Address Problems," testimony by Lawrence Thomson, May 20, 1993, GAO/T-HRD-93-24: 2.

156 Edward Wrobel, Jr., "Out of Remission?" *Emphasis* 4 (1992): 6–9.

156 Troyen Brennan et al., "Incidence of Adverse Events and Negligence in Hospitalized Patients," *New England Journal of Medicine* 324 (1991): 370–76.

156 Paul Weiler et al., "Proposal for Medical Liability Reform," *JAMA* 267 (1992): 2355–58.

156 William Johnson et al., "The Economic Consequences of Medical Injuries," *JAMA* 267 (1992): 2487–92.

157 Richard Schmitt, "Trial Lawyers Pinpoint Areas for Litigation," *Wall Street Journal*, August 9, 1993: B1.

157 David Rogers, "Initial Clinton Medical Malpractice Reform Plan Pulled After Resistance by Entrenched Interests," *Wall Street Journal*, June 15, 1993: A20.

157 Edward Wrobel, Jr., "Out of Remission?" *Emphasis* 4 (1992): 6–9.

157 A. Russell Localio et al., "Relation Between Malpractice and Adverse Events Due to Negligence," *New England Journal of Medicine* 325 (1991): 245–51.

157 Paul Weiler et al., "Proposal for Medical Liability Reform," *JAMA* 267 (1992): 2355–58.

157 Mark Taragin et al., "The Influence of Standard of Care and Severity of Injury on the Resolution of Medical Malpractice Claims," *Annals of Internal Medicine* 117 (1992): 780–784.

157 William Johnson et al., "The Economic Consequences of Medical Injuries," *JAMA* 267 (1992): 2487–92.

157 American College of Obstetricians and Gynecologists, news release, October 21, 1992.

158 American College of Obstetricians and Gynecologists, news release, October 21, 1992.

158 Kevin Sack, "Rise Granted on Insurance for Doctors," *New York Times*, July 27, 1993: B1.

158 "Medical Malpractice: Experience With Efforts to Address Problems," testimony by Lawrence Thomson, May 20, 1993, GAO/T-HRD-93-24: 16.

158 "Economic Implications of Rising Health Care Costs," Congressional Budget Office, October 1992: 27.

158 William Johnson et al., "The Economic Consequences of Medical Injuries," *JAMA* 267 (1992): 2487–92.

159 A. Russell Localio et al., "Relationship Between Malpractice Claims and Cesarean Delivery," *JAMA* 269 (1993): 366–73.

159 National Association of Insurance Commissioners, 1991 and 1992 data.

159 Sarah Lyall, "$700 Million Malpractice Insurance Fund Is Viewed as a Source of Blue Cross Aid," *New York Times*, December 26, 1992: A26.

160 Bill Clements, "Claims Against Primary Physicians Rise," *American Medical News*, September 14, 1992: 21.

160 David Azevedo, "Courts Let UR Firms Off the Hook—and Leave Doctors On," *Medical Economics*, January 25, 1993: 30–44.

161 Edward Felsenthal, "Doctors Confront Threat of Jail for Errors," *Wall Street Journal*, September 13, 1993: B3.

161 Edward Felsenthal, "Life-and-Death Medical Cases Drag in Courts," *Wall Street Journal*, February 17, 1993: B1.

162 John Ferguson et al., "Court-Ordered Reimbursement for Unproven Medical Technology," *JAMA* 269 (1993): 2116–21.

162 Linda Greenhouse, "Hospital Appeals Ruling on Treating Baby Born With Most of Brain Gone," *New York Times*, September 24, 1993: A10.

163 Jeanne Kassler, "Judge Rules AIDS Is Not VD," *Medical Tribune*, November 17, 1988: 20 (editorial).

163 "Baby Without Viable Brain Dies, But Legal Struggle Will Continue," *New York Times*, March 31, 1992: A14.

163 Tamar Lewin, "Man Is Allowed to Let Daughter Die," *New York Times*, January 27, 1993: A12.

163 Lisa Belkin, "In Right-to-Die Fight, Court Finds Family Liable for Care," *New York Times*, September 24, 1992: B6.

164 David Stipp, "Some Question Extent of Lead's Risk to Kids, Need to Remove Paint," *Wall Street Journal*, September 16, 1993: A1.

164 Richard Schmitt, "Whistles Blow More Often on Health Care," *Wall Street Journal*, September 2, 1993: B1.

164 Calvin Sims, "Blood Labs Agree to Pay $39.8 Million," *New York Times*, September 14, 1993: D1.

Part Three: What to Do

165 Lawrence Weed, *Medical Records, Medical Education, and Patient Care*, Case Western Reserve University, 1971.

Chapter 13: Principles of Reform

169 "Employer-Based Health Insurance," Government Accounting Office, GAO/HRD-92-125, September 1992: 6–7.

170 "Healthcare: Problems and Potential Lessons for Reform," Statement of Charles Bowsher, Comptroller General of the United States, GAO/T-HRD-92-23, March 27, 1992: 5.

171 Steven Miles et al., authors' reply to letters in *New England Journal of Medicine* 328 (1993): 970–71.

173 Nancy Adler et al., "Socioeconomic Inequalities in Health: No Easy Solution," *JAMA* 269 (1993): 140–45.

173 David Wessel, "Coming Federal Battle: Health Costs vs. Poor," *Wall Street Journal*, May 11, 1992: A1.

174 Timothy Egan, "Old, Ailing and Finally a Burden Abandoned," *New York Times*, March 26, 1992: A1.

174 "Chinese Reforms Linked to Illness," *Wall Street Journal*, August 3, 1993: A11.

174 James Fries, "Reducing Health Care Costs by Reducing the Need and Demand for Medical Services," *New England Journal of Medicine* 329 (1993): 321–25.

175 Louise Russell, "The Role of Prevention in Health Reform," *New England Journal of Medicine* 329 (1993): 352–54.

175 John Taylor, "Don't Blame Me," *New York Magazine*, June 3, 1991: 26–34.
176 Rick Wartzman and Hilary Stout, "Administration Critics Search Membership List of Health-Care Task Force for Goldberg, Rube," *Wall Street Journal*, June 16, 1993: A14.
177 David Himmelstein and Steffie Woolhandler, letter to the editor, *New England Journal of Medicine* 328 (1993): 1789.
178 Stephen Kreitzer, letter to the editor, *New England Journal of Medicine* 328 (1993): 1789.
178 "Emergency Departments," General Accounting Office, GAO/HRD-93-4, January 1993: 3–13.
179 Robert Fuller, "Hospitals: Debt Costs Will Rise," *New York Times*, July 25, 1993: F13.
179 John Iglehart, "The American Health Care System: Community Hospitals," *New England Journal of Medicine* 329 (1993): 372–76.
180 "Economic Implications of Rising Health Care Costs," CBO Study, October 1992: 40, 46–47.
182 Kathryn Jones, "Wal-Mart Loses Suit On Pricing," *New York Times*, October 13, 1993: D1.
182 Charles McCoy, "Foundation Health Shares Fall Sharply After Loss of Military Contract to Aetna," *Wall Street Journal*, July 30, 1993: B5.
182 "Aetna Contract on Health Care," *New York Times*, December 29, 1993: D9.
183 David Eddy, "Three Bullets to Watch in the 1990s," *JAMA* 270 (1993): 520–26.
184 Thomas Graboys et al., "Results of a Second-Opinion Trial Among Patients Recommended for Coronary Angiography," *JAMA* 268 (1992): 2537–40.
185 Michael Waldholz and Hilary Stout, "A New Debate Rages Over the Patenting of Gene Discoveries," *Wall Street Journal*, April 17, 1992: A1.
185 Norman Carey, "Ethics, Money, and the Human Genome," *BMJ* 304 (1992): 725–26.
187 "Emergency Departments," General Accounting Office, GAO/HRD-93-4, January 1993: 3–13.
187 Jennifer Haas et al., "The Effect of Health Coverage for Uninsured Pregnant Women on Maternal Health and the Use of Cesarean Section," *JAMA* 270 (1993): 61–64.
187 "Medicaid. HealthPASS: An Evaluation of a Managed Care Program for Certain Philadelphia Recipients," General Accounting Office, GAO/HRD-93-67, May 1993: 5, 6, 29.
188 George Gellert et al., "Lead Poisoning Among Low-Income Children in Orange County, California," *JAMA* 270 (1993): 69–71.
188 Nancy Adler et al., "Socioeconomic Inequalities in Health: No Easy Solution," *JAMA* 209 (1993): 3140–45.
189 Sarah Lubman, "School-Based Health Insurance for Kids Catches on as a Way to Cover Uninsured," *Wall Street Journal*, August 31, 1993: B1.
191 Burson-Marsteller, "European Health Care Trends," June 18, 1993: A12.
191 "Nurses in Japan Walk Out," *Wall Street Journal*, April 6, 1992: A12.
191 Alexander Dorozynski, "French Doctors on Protest Strike," *BMJ* 304 (1992): 1649–50.
191 Ferdinand Protzman, "Germany Approves Sweeping Health Care Reform," *New York Times*, December 20, 1992: 8.

191 Robert Blendon, "Physicians' Perspectives on Caring for Patients in the United States, Canada, and West Germany," *New England Journal of Medicine* 328 (1993): 1011–16.

192 John Iglehart, "The American Health Care System: Community Hospitals," *New England Journal of Medicine* 329 (1993): 372–76.

192 Erik Eckholm, "Study Links Paperwork to 25% of Hospital Costs," *New York Times*, August 5, 1993: A14.

192 Donald Redelmeier and Victor Fuchs, "Hospital Expenditures in the United States and Canada," *New England Journal of Medicine* 328 (1993): 772–78.

192 Philip Lee and Richard Lamm, "Europe's Medical Model," *New York Times*, March 1, 1993: A15 (op-ed).

192 Charles Bennett, "Health Care in Austria," *JAMA* 269 (1993): 2789–94.

193 Celia Hall, "Homeopathy Study Reveals 750,100 Treatments a Year," *The Independent* (Britain), December 30, 1989.

193 "Preventive Health Care for Children," General Accounting Office GAO/HRD-93-62, August 1993: 18–19.

193 John Iglehart, "Germany's Health Care System" (part 1), *New England Journal of Medicine* 324 (1991): 503–8.

193 "1993 German Health Reforms: New Cost Control Initiatives," General Accounting Office, GAO/HRD-93-103, July, 1993: 31.

193 Jonathan Fielding and Pierre-Jean Lancy, "Lessons from France—Vive la Différence," *JAMA* 270 (1993): 748–56.

194 "1993 German Health Reforms: New Cost Control Initiatives," General Accounting Office, GAO/HRD-93-103, July 1993: 22, 25–26.

194 Michael Whitcomb and J. P. Desgroseilliers, "Primary Care Medicine in Canada," *New England Journal of Medicine* 326 (1992): 1469–72.

195 Craig Whitney, "Health Care Evolves as Issue in Britain's General Election," *New York Times*, March 28, 1992: I1.

195 John Iglehart, "Germany's Health Care System" (part 2), *New England Journal of Medicine* 324 (1991): 1750–56.

195 Susan Dentzer, "Looking for *Wa*," *Dartmouth Medicine*, Summer 1992: 21–26.

195 John Iglehart, "Health Systems in Three Nations," *Health Affairs*, Fall 1991: 259.

196 Kevin Grumbach and John Fry, "Managing Primary Care in the United States and in the United Kingdom," *New England Journal of Medicine* 328 (1993): 940–45.

196 "Robots for the Operating Room," *New York Times*, July 19, 1992: F9.

196 David Taylor, "Prescribing in Europe—Forces for Change," *BMJ* 304 (1992): 239–42.

196 Susan Dentzer, "Looking for *Wa*," *Dartmouth Medicine*, Summer 1992: 20, 21–26.

196 John Danaher, "Health Care in Japan: A Cultural Odessey," *Dartmouth Medicine*, Summer 1992: 27.

196 John Danaher, "A Cultural Odessey," *Dartmouth Medicine*, Summer 1992: 27–29.

197 Susan Dentzer, "Looking for *Wa*," *Dartmouth Medicine*, Summer 1992: 22–23.

197 David Taylor, "Prescribing in Europe—Forces for Change," *BMJ* 304 (1992): 239–42.

197 Charles Bennett, "Health Care in Austria," *JAMA* 269 (1993): 2789–94.
197 Edward Felsenthal, "Maine Limits Liability for Doctors Who Meet Treatment Guidelines," *Wall Street Journal*, April 3, 1993: A1.
197 "Medical Malpractice: Experience With Efforts to Address Problems," testimony by Lawrence Thomson, May 20, 1993, GAO/T-HRD-93-24: 2.
198 Edward Felsenthal, "Maine Limits Liability for Doctors Who Meet Treatment Guidelines," *Wall Street Journal*, April 3, 1993: A1.
198 Medical Malpractice: Experience With Efforts to Address Problems," testimony by Lawrence Thomson, May 20, 1993, GAO/T-HRD-93-24: 10, 11.
199 William Hsiao et al., "Assessing the Implementation of Physician-Payment Reform," *New England Journal of Medicine* 328 (1993): 928–33.
199 George Anders and Ron Winslow, "Health-Care Industry Is Now Restructuring; With It Comes Pain," *Wall Street Journal*, June 16, 1993: A1.
199 George Anders, "Rx for Sales," *Wall Street Journal*, September 10, 1993: A1.
199 Victor Fuchs, "Dear President Clinton," *JAMA* 269 (1993): 1678–79.
200 Artin Mahmoudi and Michael Iseman, "Pitfalls in the Care of Patients With Tuberculosis," *JAMA* 270 (1993): 65–68.
201 "Medical Malpractice: Experience With Efforts to Address Problems," testimony by Lawrence Thomson, May 20, 1993, GAO/T-HRD-93-24: 12.
202 David Rogers, "Initial Clinton Malpractice Reform Plan Pulled After Resistance by Entrenched Interests," *Wall Street Journal*, June 15, 1993: A20.
202 Kevin Salwen, "Tax Credit to Increase Hiring of Poor Is Found by U.S. Official to Waste Funds," *Wall Street Journal*, August 24, 1993: A2.
202 "Taxes Curb Smoking," *Wall Street Journal*, September 1, 1993: A1.
203 "1993 German Health Reforms," General Accounting Office, GAO/HRD-93-103, July 1993: 16.

Epilogue

206 "Health Insurance: California Public Employees' Alliance Has Reduced Recent Premium Growth," General Accounting Office, GAO/HRD-94-40, November 1993: 1–19.
208 Kevin Anderson, personal communication, October 29, 1993.

Index

231